The Homeopathic Miasms

A Modern View

The Homeopathic Miasms

A Modern View

by Ian Watson

Cutting Edge Publications
Totnes
Devon
England

First published in the United Kingdom 2009

Cutting Edge Publications
PO Box 156
Totnes
Devon
TQ9 6ZP
England

www.cuttingedgepublications.co.uk

A catalogue record for this book is available from the British Library

ISBN 978-0-9517657-8-4

Other Works by Ian Watson

Books ~ www.cuttingedgepublications.co.uk

A Guide to the Methodologies of Homeopathy
Aspects of Homeopathy: *Musculo-Skeletal Problems*
The Tao of Homeopathy

Recordings ~ www.ianwatsondownloads.com

A Remedy for Everything
A Remedy for Everything Else
Becoming a Confident Prescriber
Casetaking & Case Analysis
Cycles, Seasons, Ages & Stages
Dynamic Homeopathy
Dynamic Materia Medica
Flower Essences for Homeopaths
Health & The Planets
Homeopathy & The Chakras
Homeopathy: Transitional Medicine
Living Abundantly
Mental & Emotional Health
Musculo-Skeletal Problems
Organ Remedies
Running a Successful Practice
Seven Herbs
Shadow Work
Skin Problems: Healing from Within
The Alchemy of Personal Change
The Healing Journey
The Inner Work Series
The Natural Traveler
The Quest for Wholeness
The Tao of Homeopathy
Therapeutics & Layers
Understanding the Miasms

Contents

Introduction

This book began life as a series of lectures and discussions which took place in various locations during a three–year period. Having formulated the initial ideas, I was eager to share them with other homeopaths in order to obtain feedback, but I also had some anxiety as to the kind of feedback I might receive!

By a stroke of good fortune, an opportunity presented for me to give my very first talk on the subject to a group of homeopathic students in Iceland. I figured that if the feedback was unfavourable, at least it would take a while for it to reach the wider homeopathic community. As it turned out, the material was enthusiastically received and the students encouraged me to develop the ideas further with the input and assistance of many subsequent individuals and groups.

The main body of this work grew out of a gradual realization that the miasm theory developed by Hahnemann contained a built–in limitation. It was a long time before I was able to articulate what I considered the nature of this limitation to be, although I was well aware of its effects, namely to encourage homeopaths to think and to act allopathically.

It became apparent to me that when we refer to some invisible entity which is transmitted from one person to another, infecting them and causing sickness, we have adopted an allopathic attitude. Similarly, when we prescribe remedies with the intention of carrying out 'anti–miasmatic' treatment, that is really no different to the intention behind the prescription of antibiotics. I do not believe that this approach is wrong, or even unhelpful, but it does have its limitations.

Having acknowledged that this is the case, I decided to attempt to develop a new way of looking at the chronic miasms which included positive as well as negative traits, and to view them as transformative influences that could be understood, learned from and integrated, rather than as disease–producing forces that needed to be subdued or eradicated. I trust that the ideas presented here go some way in that direction.

As the work took shape, I decided to include some information on the nosodes and major remedies associated with each miasm, to prevent it from becoming too abstract and to demonstrate its practical value as an aid to both learning and prescribing. I have expanded this part of the book to include some suggestions on the use of flower essences for the issues that I have come to associate with each of the major miasms.

I am aware that during the intervening years between my original lectures on this topic and the completion of this book, a number of new volumes on the miasms have been published by different authors. I have deliberately avoided studying any of them until now, and am looking forward to discovering if any common threads are to be found.

I would like to thank Carol Nelson for transcribing my original recorded material on this subject, and Nevine Fathy for assembling it into a format more suitable for publication.

Ian Watson
Devon, U.K. 2009

The Miasm Theory

The miasmatic theory of disease was formulated and refined by Hahnemann during the latter part of his long and fruitful life. As was his custom, he tailored the new theory to match his actual clinical experience. We can deduce from his writings in *The Organon* and *Chronic Diseases* that he was inspired to create the concept of miasms for two main reasons.

First, it provided an explanation as to why, even after proper homeopathic treatment and removal of any external maintaining causes, there remained an underlying tendency towards disease which seemed to continue unchecked throughout an individual's life. Second, and more importantly, it gave practitioners a radical new reason for prescribing which, by shifting the principle of similars onto another level, enabled previously incurable patients to become amenable to cure by homeopathic means.

Prior to the adoption of the miasm theory, homeopaths could only conceive of matching a similar remedy to the existing state that each patient presented, and when a new symptom–picture emerged, a fresh similar remedy was selected. Whilst this method continued to hold good, the miasm theory allowed, and indeed required, that remedies could also be matched to the underlying predisposition towards disease that manifests throughout a person's life in various different forms.

This was a momentous shift, and history shows that many of Hahnemann's contemporaries were unable to make the leap in understanding that he had made, thus rejecting or simply ignoring the miasmatic theory. Nonetheless, the theory took hold because it proved its practical value to those who put it to the test. Any practitioner who observes the results obtained in cases of long–term sickness, as did Hahnemann, finds that there are indeed underlying predispositions towards disease, that they can be classified under general headings as he suggested, and that the tendencies themselves can be prescribed upon to the greater benefit of the patient.

Homeopaths now had the means to treat, for example, acute hay fever during the summer months, and to treat the pre–existing inherited tendency to hay fever once the acute phase had subsided. J.T. Kent remarked in one of his lectures that only when he understood the sycotic basis of asthma was he able to feel confident about curing the condition rather than only temporarily palliating it.

We know from Rima Handley's translations of Hahnemann's case notes that during the latter stage of his life he was prescribing *Sulphur* to around ninety percent of his patients, without it being the most similar remedy, so it is clear that he was prescribing it for a different reason. Hahnemann, we must remember, was a dedicated empiricist and he was evidently very good at breaking his own rules.

Hahnemann had found that the only way to get a sense of the underlying state was to record all of the ailments his patients had suffered throughout their entire lives, even taking into account the family history. He thus built up the picture of each miasm systematically by taking the case histories of hundreds of people.

It was a similar process to the one he had developed for conducting a proving of a newly-discovered remedy, and for deducing the *genus epidemicus* in acute conditions, where each individual case manifests only a small part of the total picture. People who were chronically sick were seen to be manifesting only a small portion of the miasmatic picture. To perceive the whole, it is necessary to piece the individual parts together like a jigsaw puzzle.

Hahnemann came to the conclusion that it was perfectly acceptable to give the indicated remedies based on the presenting symptoms, and also to simultaneously prescribe on the miasmatic tendency behind the symptoms, using a quite different remedy. This gave rise to a whole new classification of certain remedies which became known as *'anti-miasmatics'*.

My own experience in homeopathic practice demonstrated to me that Hahnemann was right. If you don't treat an active miasm with the appropriate nosode or miasmatic remedy, eventually you will notice that people apparently get well, but there remains an underlying tendency that isn't cured. After a while, you perceive a relapse or recurrence of health problems, or the disease manifests in a slightly different form. One thing clears up, only for something else to appear. These, according to Hahnemann, are manifestations of the same underlying miasmatic tendency, and are not to be viewed as separate diseases.

Development of the Miasm Theory

Contemporary practitioners have, in light of their experience, developed the miasm theory further along the lines established by Hahnemann. It was observed over time that certain disease phenomena which were becoming prevalent in practice could not be adequately encompassed within the three original miasmatic categories of psora, sycosis and syphilis. Within Hahnemann's lifeteime, a fourth miasm named 'pseudo-psora' was postulated to embrace disease states not covered by the existing trio, and eventually this came to be recognized as the tuberculosis miasm.

More recently, the cancer miasm has come to be widely recognised and accepted. Other chronic miasms have been suggested in the last few decades but have not yet gained the widespread acceptance of the 'big five'. Some of these new miasms will be discussed at the end of this book.

The other main development in the application of the miasm theory has been in the widespread use of the major nosodes. Traditionally, homeopaths favoured the use of similar remedies that were known to have a close relationship with each miasm. Hahnemann recommended *Sulphur* as the leading anti-psoric, *Thuja* for sycosis and *Mercurius* for syphilis, although we know from his case–notes that he also experimented with an early form of *Psorinum*, which he named *Psoricum*.

The clinical uses of the other nosodes were developed chiefly by Drs. J.C. Burnett, J.H. Clarke, T. Skinner and H.C. Allen among others. The researches of these homeopaths gave us the remedy pictures of *Medorrhinum*, *Syphilinum* and *Tuberculinum*. We are also indebted to Dr. Donald Foubister, whose relatively recent observations enabled *Carcinosin* to join the ranks of the polychrests.

Some homeopaths argue that the nosodes are just like any

other remedy that should only be prescribed when indicated on the symptom picture. Other homeopaths have developed an irrational fear of the nosodes, and refuse to prescribe them even when indicated.

My own experience taught me that nosodes can often do things in a chronic case that the other remedies cannot do. All of the successful homeopaths that I've had the good fortune to study and work with have used nosodes extensively in their practice, and I've met a few practitioners who used very little else.

It is clear, then, that the practical applications of the miasm theory have continued to multiply and develop, but what of the theory itself? The basic tenets that we inherited from Hahnemann have remained virtually unchanged since his death, and it is these that I would like to explore in the following two chapters.

Hahnemann's View of the Miasms

As was stated earlier, Hahnemann held the view that there existed three chronic miasms which he named psora, sycosis and syphilis. Each miasm he held to be responsible for a range of disease phenomena. The psoric, which he affectionately termed *'that thousand-headed monster'* was credited with producing seven-eighths of all chronic pathologies. The sycotic and syphilitic were held jointly responsible for the remaining eighth.

Hahnemann went to considerable lengths to document the ailments associated with each miasm, and to suggest treatment plans for their eradication. What he did not elaborate upon were the questions that have often puzzled me: what is the true nature and purpose of the miasms? Why do they produce only suffering for humankind? Is homeopathy really the only means by which miasms can be treated, as Hahnemann asserts? Might the miasms have some positive or beneficial aspects from which we could learn something?

In order to address these questions, it is first necessary to understand in greater depth the perspective from which Hahnemann was writing when he recorded his new theory in the early 1800's.

While the miasmatic theory was taking shape in Hahnemann's mind, Edward Jenner (1749–1823) and other pioneers were simultaneously making observations based on their own experiences, which were to lead to the development of the germ theory of disease and the use of vaccines as a form of prophylaxis. That Hahnemann was influenced by these discoveries within allopathy is beyond question—he comments upon them directly in *The Organon* and in *Chronic Diseases*. What is not so well acknowledged amongst homeopaths is the extent to which the miasm theory is in fact analagous to the emerging germ theory.

6

In the lengthy introduction to his *Chronic Diseases*, for example, Hahnemann uses the terms *infection, infectious, contagion* and *contagious* to describe the way in which miasms may be transmitted from one individual to another. In his introduction he compares the curative process to the army of a country, which *'drives the enemy out'*, and talks of *'these hostile powers which produce disease and against which the vital force alone is no match'*.

He goes on to describe these disease–producing influences as the *'invading morbific enemy'* which lurks in the body and uses the terms *parasitic* and *parasitical* on numerous occasions. In *Chronic Diseases* he describes how *'infection'* with a chronic miasm occurs in a single moment, but a period of latency follows before any outward symptoms become manifest, just as was found to occur with infectious diseases.

Whilst allowing for the possibility that some mistranslation of terms has occurred, it seems certain that Hahnemann made some very similar assumptions about miasms as allopathic medical science would make about bacteria and viruses.

Hahnemann's context for understanding the miasms may be summarised as follows:

(i) Miasms are invisible malevolent forces, each of which creates a range of suffering of a particular kind
Each miasm, most especially the psoric, has a huge spectrum of disease states associated with it. No individual can manifest the whole miasmatic state at once, therefore the disease–image of a miasm has to be built up from observation of many cases, in much the same way as a remedy–picture is built up from many provers.

(ii) Miasms are wholly negative influences which need to be eradicated
As far as I am aware, Hahnemann doesn't have a good word

to say about any of the miasms. His writings are focused exclusively on the diseases that each miasm produces, and the remedies needed to remove those diseases. This orientation towards disease has permeated virtually everything that has been written about the miasms since Hahnemann's death.

(iii) Miasms are transmitted from one person to another by inheritance, sexual contact or (in the case of psora) merely by close proximity or touch

Hahnemann's description of the ways in which miasms may be transmitted from one person to another show a marked similarity to the allopathic model of infectious disease transmission. In relation to psora, he writes that infection can occur from such circumstances as *'touching the general skin; the physician feeling the pulse; wearing new gloves which had been tried on by another; staying in a strange lodging place; using a strange towel for drying oneself; a babe from the caresses of its nurse or a stranger; and thousands of other possible ways'* (Chronic Diseases page 79–80). He adds that the syphilitic and sycotic miasms generally require genital contact in order that contagion takes place.

(iv) The innate self-healing capacity of the human organism is unable of its own accord to overcome the negative morbific influence of the miasms

Despite his inherent faith in the ability of the vital force to maintain a healthy state, Hahnemann seems to have concluded that the diseases resulting from the chronic miasms were an exception to the rule. This is in contradiction to acute diseases, which he observed to have a natural tendency towards self-resolution.

(v) Anti-miasmatic homeopathic treatment is necessary in order to *'drive out the enemy'* of miasm-induced disease

If miasms are perceived as morbific influences, against which the vital principle is unable to re–establish a state of health, then it follows that homeopathic treatment *against* the miasms will be justified and necessary. What seems to have been overlooked by successive generations of homeopaths is that this mode of treatment is essentially allopathic, the only difference being the type of medicines employed.

Reading these early writings, I began to realize that the miasmatic theory in its original form is really a branch of allopathic thinking hidden within homeopathy. This is an area in which we homeopaths become allopaths without realizing it. We forget about treating the person and instead we want to get rid of the miasm. Hence, the miasm theory has a serious limitation built into it. It works up to a point, just as the germ theory of disease does, but it is not a particularly holistic view of health and disease.

The Kentian Perspective

James Tyler Kent embraced the miasm theory wholeheartedly, and added a moralistic dimension that surpasses anything you will find in the writings of Hahnemann. As a disciple of the Christian mystic Emanuel Swedenborg (1688–1772), Kent held the view that the miasms and all the misery they brought to humankind were the natural result of the degraded moral state into which human beings had fallen. *'Psora,'* he wrote, *'is the evolution of the state of man's will, the ultimates of sin.'* In one of his famous quotes, he states that *'The human race today walking the face of the earth is but little better than a moral leper.'* (J.T. Kent, *Lectures on Homeopathic Philosophy*).

This association between what Kent calls *'Willing evils..... thinking that which is false'* and the psoric miasm has become a persistent idea in the collective homeopathic consciousness, and the link between psora and the Christian doctrine of 'original sin' has been endorsed and reinforced by many other homeopathic sources.

In a similar vein, Kent picks up the social stigma attached to the venereal diseases gonorrhoea and syphilis, and carries it across to the corresponding sycotic and syphilitic miasms. In his *Lectures*, he says *'If we look upon syphilis we will see that man's own act leads him to the place where he comes in contact with syphilis; it is the result of action......syphilis is that disease which corresponds to the effect of impure coition, of going where syphilis is, of coming in contact with those who have it........it is an action; it is not so with psora.'*

Kent seemed to be of the opinion that if humans would only rectify their wrong thinking and curb their destructive behavioural habits, then miasms would cease to be a problem. While I find his conclusions to be somewhat idealistic, I would still give Kent the credit for attempting to elevate the miasm theory to another level. He says, *'The susceptibility to psora opens out a question altogether too broad to study among the sciences in a medical college. It is altogether too extensive, for it goes to the very primitive wrong of the human race, the very first sickness of the human race, that is, the spiritual sickness.'*

If we overlook the moral tone, we can see that Kent was ahead of his time in recognizing *the state of human consciousness* as being fundamental to understanding what the miasmatic energies are really about, and this is the theme I would like to develop in the following chapters.

Re-Considering the Miasms

Although Hahnemann was ahead of his time in considering individual susceptibility and the energetic basis of disease, his context for the miasms was nonetheless based on the prevailing medical model of the early 1800's. The miasm was considered to be something 'out there' with which people become infected, it makes them sick, it spreads via 'contagion' and we have to wage a war against this invisible enemy in order to combat the diseases it produces. If this sounds all too familiar, there is a good reason.

Homeopaths are justified in pointing out the obvious limitations of the allopathic germ theory, and we witness all too readily how a treatment that is based upon this theory, such as antibiotics, does not satisfy the highest ideals of cure. Similarly, I would argue that the miasm theory as Hahnemann left it has exactly the same limitations, and these will only be overcome if we can revise and expand the theory to include a more holistic perspective.

In the existing miasmatic model, there is a built–in dependence on the experts with the specialist 'anti–miasmatic' medicines which is, I believe, burdensome for practitioners and disempowering for patients. That homeopaths discovered the miasms, and are the only ones who have the technology to treat them is a viewpoint that makes people totally dependent on homeopathy and powerless to participate in their own self–healing.

Personally, I no longer believe that homeopathy has a monopoly on miasmatic treatment, nor do I believe that miasms are something to be gotten rid of per se. I would like to introduce the idea that miasms can be addressed and also understood in a number of different ways, and that this new understanding will enhance the experience of both practitioners and their patients. My understanding is that, in nature, everything has its equal and opposite. Nothing is wholly good or wholly bad, including what we call disease, and I assume that the same is true of the miasms.

Some years ago, I started to consider what else the miasms could bring to humankind apart from the disease aspects. We can look at disease itself as a growth opportunity, for example, or as the organism's best attempt to heal itself. One way we can empower ourselves in the treatment of disease is to embrace it as something which informs us about our lifestyle, tendencies, habit patterns, and emotional behavior. We can begin to consider the possibility that we *participated* in the creation of this problem, rather than holding to the victim position that something 'out there' is doing it to us.

It occurred to me that it might be interesting to attempt to view the miasms as *opportunities* rather than as enemies. If they have a negative pole, they must also have a positive pole. Hahnemann and Kent gave us the negative side of the miasms. I adopted the position of considering each miasm as a *neutral* energetic influence, which could have both positive and negative effects, depending on the circumstance and the response to it. This is not an easy position to maintain when you are working with terms like cancer and syphilis, but it can be done.

I also tried to clarify some of the basic life issues that each miasm represents, in order to get an understanding of why, for example, sycosis has an affinity with the mucus membranes, growths and genitalia. Why does syphilis have an affinity with bones, ulceration and destruction of tissue? These associations are well–established in the homeopathic literature, but I have not come across an explanation of these relationships that made any sense to me.

Focusing on the life issues, affinities and themes of the miasms rather than the disease processes presents an opportunity to engage with them in a participatory way. You have a choice to see the miasm as an influence you can work with, learn from and be transformed by, rather than as something that is attacking you that has to be driven out.

As a practitioner, if you can grasp the issues of the miasm in a neutral sense, then the diseases as well as the positive potentialities become relatively easy to figure out and understand. You can also look at the key features of a remedy you haven't studied before, and understand that remedy miasmatically by knowing its affinities and the issues that both the remedy and the miasm represent.

In the following chapters I will cover the 'big five' chronic miasms in some detail from this neutral perspective. I have also made some tentative suggestions regarding several of the newer miasms and the life issues they relate to at the end of the book.

As an illustration of how we can work with miasmatic influences in a more participatory way, I have included some material on flower essences that can be related to the core themes of each miasm. Flower essences do not have the orientation towards 'curing disease' that is found in the great bulk of homeopathic literature. Rather, they are concerned with facilitating a transformation of consciousness in both practitioner and patient. As such, they are ideally suited to working with miasms as agents of transformation and inner growth.

Psora
Survival on Planet Earth

I began by thinking of psora as the first challenge to humanity, and then I attempted to look at each of the other major miasms as a subsequent challenge. I tried to imagine that I had just arrived on planet earth among the first humans, and began to explore what effect this would have on my consciousness. I came to the rather obvious conclusion that immediate survival needs would be the first challenge to humanity, and I feel that this is what the psoric miasm really represents.

What is it that threatens our immediate survival on planet earth? Temperature, weather, animals, accidents, injuries, warriors, being attacked, acute disease, and a lack of adequate nutrition and water. Something we humans have in common with all living things is a tendency to protect ourselves, to keep ourselves alive by finding sufficient food and water and amenable living conditions in which to thrive. That tendency, which is pre-programmed and almost entirely instinctual, is what psora could actually be about—the *tendency to self-survival*. Adaptation to a hostile landscape and changing climate, securing a regular supply of clean water and nutritious food, these are the realities we have to accept in order to thrive on planet earth.

First of all, our body has to adapt to the change in the seasons. The process of transition, when one season turns into another, is a time when many people get ill. If we mal-adapt, if we fail to meet the challenge of psora adequately, we get sick with diseases that would be called 'psoric' in homeopathy. It has to do with being out of alignment with natural cycles. Something similar occurs when we fly across the world and find ourselves dropped into a different climate zone where we have to make a sudden adjustment to a drastic change in our outer environment.

If we are aligned with nature, we tend to live more simply and also more seasonally. We might hibernate to some degree during the winter months, for example, and eat the foods that are locally available at each time of year. If the springtime brings the urge to clear out our clutter and 'spring clean' the house, we should follow it, because these instinctual impulses are linking us back to the natural world.

Nutrition is clearly a very important part of this challenge. Hahnemann was as much a naturopath as a homeopath, although this aspect of his work is largely ignored today. When he wrote about maintaining causes and obstacles to cure, which he frequently did, he was often talking about diet and living conditions that were contributing to, if not causing, numerous diseases.

In our modern Western culture we have too much food of too little quality. The nutritional value of our food has been degraded through industrial–scale growing and processing methods, and the produce itself has been irradiated and contaminated with pesticides, herbicides, preservatives and such like. We are eating foods which are grown out of season and transported across vast distances, creating a further rupture in our ever–diminishing connection to the natural world.

Fortunately, people all over the world are now waking up to the ecological and health crisis that we ourselves have created by neglecting to pay attention to the most basic psoric reality. There is a natural order to life on this beautiful planet of ours, and we neglect to pay attention to this fact at our own peril.

The Psoric Challenges

Temperature
A common theme amongst the so–called 'antipsoric' remedies is that they tend to have issues around temperature. They are either too hot or too cold, or they have alternations between the two. If you consider for a moment the king and queen of psora, *Sulphur* and *Psorinum*. *Sulphur* is typically boiling hot, sticks his feet out of bed, gets easily overheated and wears a tee shirt in the winter, whilst *Psorinum* wears a thick coat and hat in the summer and can never get warm enough.

All of the main psoric remedies have the same theme of mal–adaptation to temperature or climate which, as we have already mentioned, is one of the basic survival issues that we are faced with.

Hunger
The psoric remedies also have a problem with appetite and hunger. The archetypal psoric duo *Sulphur* and *Psorinum* are two of the hungriest remedies in the materia medica. They have a weak, empty feeling at eleven in the morning *(Sulph.)*, the stomach starts to rumble, the person feels weak and they have to eat something, so we have problems with the blood sugar and a tendency towards hypoglycaemia.

When we're in harmony with our biological rhythms, we eat when we're hungry, drink when we're thirsty, sleep when we're tired, work when we're awake and active, and so on. We don't have to think about it. When we're out of alignment, these patterns get confused. We have just eaten, and half an hour later, we're hungry again, like *Lycopodium* and *Sulphur*. Or we become hungry at inappropriate times. *Psorinum* has to get up in the middle of the night and raid the fridge, or the person gets hungry with a headache, not necessarily because they need to eat.

Metabolism

Nutrition, and the processes of assimilation (taking in what we need to maintain health and to grow and repair our bodies) and elimination (getting rid of those things we don't need) are part of the psoric pattern. Assimilation and elimination need to be in balance. Major psoric remedies such as *Lycopodium, Sulphur,* and *Psorinum* are on the fast metabolic side. No matter how much they eat, it never feels quite enough and they are hungry again in a very short time. The *Calcarea* group and *Graphites* are slow metabolizers by comparison. However little they eat, they can't process it fast enough, so they gain weight easily. Or we have remedies like *Silica* and *Magnesium–carbonicum* that are unable to take sufficient nutrition from their diet because the assmilation is poor.

Elimination

Elimination is another major theme to be found amongst the psoric remedies. They tend towards constipation or diarrhea or an alternation or combination of the two, as can be seen in *Alumina, Calcarea–carbonica, Bryonia, Sulphur, Psorinum, Graphites, Nux–vomica* and many others. When the internal organs of elimination are not functioning adequately, the body recruits a reserve organ of elimination—the skin. When the liver or colon are sluggish, we tend to see increased elimination through the skin, and many of the skin problems for which psora is famous can be understood in this context.

The skin also features strongly in psora because it is our interface with what appears to be the outside world. The skin is our sensory organ for temperature, heat and cold, wet and dry. Skin disorders very often reflect mal–adaptation to temperature or environment, and they can also reflect a sense of unease with one's place in the world. We talk about being 'happy in our skin,' or 'jumping out of our skin' in response to a survival threat, which again is a psoric issue (fright). Chronic skin problems, historically, represent one of the biggest challenges to homeopaths and indeed to any system of therapy.

The major psoric remedies also have a tendency to putrefaction and offensiveness, which is a signal of poor elimination and inner toxicity. In nature, when liquids are in a state of stagnation instead of flow, offensiveness results. *Psorinum* is reputedly so offensive that you cannot stand the smell in the room. Homeopaths generally consider *Sulphur* and *Psorinum* to be the two dirtiest remedies in the materia medica. *Sulphur* is known as the 'great unwashed', and *Psorinum* is the 'great unwashable'. That takes us to the next theme, which relates to hygiene.

Hygiene

Originally, hygiene had a broader meaning than it does today, and related to all kinds of living habits that contributed to staying healthy and preventing disease. The Greek gods Asclepius and Hygeia were viewed as equal and opposite complementaries. The role of Hygeia was to promote and maintain health and the role of Asclepius was to cure disease. Modern medicine has been focusing on the interventionist, Asclepian side of medicine almost exclusively. The Hygeian side, where people learn what they must do for themselves in order to maintain their health, is now making a timely comeback.

The Hygeia aspect of health is also part of the psoric challenge. We stay healthy by maintaing reasonable standards of cleanliness, by learning how to preserve foods effectively, by ensuring we have a good balance of nutrients in our diet, by exercising regularly, and by living in conditions which are conducive to health. As best we can, we must avoid living in damp basements, unsanitary or overcrowded conditions, just as we must guard against ingesting toxins or living on junk food if we are to prevent the psoric ailments from developing.

Psora in Modern Society

We may well imagine that our immediate survival is not threatened on a daily basis now in the way it was when we were cavemen and women, but try crossing a busy road in a major city! Our immediate survival can still be threatened on a daily basis, or at least *it feels like it can*. These threats, whether real or imaginary, trigger the fight–or–flight response. The adrenal glands kick in, the heart rate increases, the blood supply gets redirected, and we're ready to fight or flee in an instant. This type of energy is related to the base or root chakra.

A chronic over–stimulation of the fight–or–flight mechanism, or living on adrenalin goes together with the psoric imbalance. This is very common in modern cities where we live as though our survival is threatened, even if it isn't. The price for that is burn–out, chronic fatigue, adrenal exhaustion, hyperactivity and low energy states. All of the psoric remedies have this problem with the base chakra energy, which governs the basic will to live and the energy to function in life.

When you feel that your energy is depleted, you will tend to crave caffeine, sugar and other stimulants, and then you may need a sleeping pill to help you sleep at night. Urban life tends to encourage a fast–food mentality, excessively long working hours, inadequate sleep and a general disturbance of our natural rhythms. It is no surprise, then, that the so-called psoric diseases are still extremely widespread even amongst those of us fortunate to be living in relatively comfortable conditions.

Mental & Emotional Aspects of Psora

Anxiety about Health/Poverty

Psoric remedies all tend to worry about their health. *Calcarea-carbonica* worries about heart disease, *Arsenicum* might worry about cancer, *Psorinum* despairs they will never get well, but they all share the same issue. Why should that be a concern? From the perspective of the caveman or cavewoman within each of us, ill health means that we can't look after our survival needs properly.

When we're sick or incapacitated for some reason, it puts us in touch with the primitive fear that we may not be able to meet our survival needs. Anxiety about health, fear of poverty or business failure runs right through *Psorinum*. In modern society you will see these same issues manifesting during periods of economic recession, when people are living in fear of losing their jobs and being unable to meet their financial commitments.

Not Enoughness

When we are out of harmony in our way of life, we develop a sense of 'not enoughness,' and this is a theme of the psoric remedies. There's not enough food, so they are always hungry. There's not enough clothing or heat, they are always chilly. There's not enough money, work, or time, or they are not healthy enough. They are not sleeping enough or they don't have enough energy.

In many cases, this is clearly a sign of an internal, psychological disturbance, because there actually is enough. Our survival needs *are* being taken care of (because we're here!), but it feels as though they might be taken away any minute. So we might start to stockpile food, money and other 'necessities'. We become hoarders. We exhaust ourselves working harder than we need to. That lack of trust that we will *continue* to survive and to be provided for is also part of the psoric miasm picture.

21

Existential Issues

One of the basic insecurities reflected very strongly in the psoric remedies is a fear about death. In *Psorinum* you also see fears about salvation. What happens to the soul after death? This is a *Sulphur–Psorinum–Calcarea* pre-occupation. Little children may start to ask, *'What happens to us when we die?'* It goes beyond that to *'How did we get here? What are we doing here? Where did we come from? Where are we going to? What does it all mean?'* These are the psoric questions. You could call it the existential miasm. It raises the existential questions that we all have, either on a conscious or subconscious level.

Abandoned/Forsaken

Something that had always puzzled me about *Psorinum* was its appearance in the repertory in bold type in the rubric *Forsaken Feeling*. As far as I could determine, *Psorinum* doesn't have the forsaken feeling in the same way that *Pulsatilla* or *Stramonium* has it, that sense of having been abandoned by one's mother or partner, for example. When I started thinking of psora as the existential miasm, only then could I really make sense of that symptom.

It seems that we are born, on an unconscious level, with a feeling of separation or alienation from our source. I think of it as part of the psoric challenge that goes together with incarnation on the earth plane. We take on the appearance of separation, and it's a pretty good illusion, because for all intents and purposes it looks and feels as though we are separate. In some stage of our life, or in one of our lifetimes, we embark on a journey to reconnect with that original knowledge that we are actually a part of the entire cosmos. We become aware that this connection was always there, but we couldn't see it at the time.

This re–awakening to our spiritual dimension is associated, I believe, with the tubercular miasm, and will be discussed later in the book. In the meantime, we may suffer with a niggling, background anxiety that we are helpless and alone in this vast, frightening place.

Homeopathic *Anacardium* can have that feeling of alienation very strongly, and *Androctonus* (scorpion) also, to an extreme degree. *Androctonus* is a great survival issue remedy, with a feeling of it being 'me against the rest of the world.' Jeremy Sherr, who introduced the remedy into homeopathy, described the scorpion type as the 'lone fighter in the desert', and suggested that Saddam Hussein would have been a likely candidate.

Addressing the Psoric Challenge

As I began to view the miasms differently, I found that I had changed my relationship to the diseases that are associated with the miasms. I could no longer see skin problems and other psoric ailments as something just to be gotten rid of. I began to see them as a reflection of the fact that the person is grappling with a psoric challenge in some area of their life.

If a person came along with predominantly psoric health problems, I would ask myself, *'Where in this person's life are they struggling with a psoric challenge? Where do they feel that their basic survival needs are threatened and not being met? Where is it that they feel they don't have enough? Where is the anxiety that they suspect that everything may be taken away? Where is the basic existential insecurity manifesting?'*

Sometimes I would give a homeopathic remedy to address the physical level and one or more flower essences to address the consciousness level as appropriate. I try to let the patients tell me what they need, rather than me deciding on their behalf. If I see someone get better and then relapse, or if something gets better but something different appears, or if the person keeps needing the same remedy over a prolonged period, I would try to identify what predisposes them to keep getting stuck in a certain way.

I found in my own practice that when a shift in consciousness seemed to be required, flower essences could catalyze that shift much more quickly than homeopathy alone could do. The homeopathic nosodes, by comparison, will often lessen a tendency to a recurrent *physical* disorder, such as hay fever every spring, asthma attacks, migraines or an allergic reaction of some kind.

It is important to emphasize that I'm not talking about getting rid of something. That is still a kind of *anti* treatment. The more we try to get rid of something, the more it will keep coming back at us. That is part of the perspective shift that I found is necessary. Because we are raised in an allopathic culture, most people who come to us operate from the belief that disease is something bad that has to be removed.

In homeopathy, we tend to think that a remedy–state is also something to be gotten rid of, whereas it might be that at least some of these states are archetypal in form, suggesting that finding an appropriate way to relate to this pattern is what is required.

Rajan Sankaran introduced the idea that every remedy picture is a response to a certain life situation. He called this *situational materia medica*. The presenting picture is viewed as the best that a person can do in the given circumstances. Perhaps, with the help of treatment, they can do something different, but we have to acknowledge that they are doing their best, and that the symptom–picture they present is both meaningful and purposeful.

I have had to expand my definition of what *perceiving what has to be cured* means to me in practice. Sometimes it means perceiving what is behind the presenting problem. It may be a belief, an attitude, a self–esteem issue or a lifestyle, and these are things that cannot really be 'cured' in the normal sense of the word. Carl Jung held the view that patients don't really get 'cured' as much as they outgrow an earlier stage and literally 'move on' when they are ready and willing to do so.

Psoric tendencies are present within all of us. All we need are the right circumstances to wake them up. If you don't believe me, I suggest you take a trip to a far and distant land, where you don't speak the language, the food tastes strange and the climate is not what you are used to. Traveling alone to India with a backpack and very little money gave me a rapid introduction to the psoric challenge, and brought up all the anxieties that I have described above, together with a representative sample of the physical ailments associated with the miasm also.

I would say that this is true of all of the miasms—they are ever–present within us, ready to be activated in response to a particular circumstance or a certain stage in our life. It's not that one culture has a certain miasm and another one doesn't. Certain challenges are more prevalent in some cultures than in others, but the fact remains that no matter how civilized or sophisticated a society becomes, those underlying psoric survival issues are never too far from the surface.

We can see it as a built–in feedback mechanism teaching us how we need to adapt ourselves to what is going on around us and also within us. I view the miasms as neutral teachers. If we listen and learn from them, perhaps we won't have to suffer as much with the so-called miasmatic diseases.

Flower Essences for the Psoric Miasm

Australian Bush Flower Essences

Old Man Banksia is a good support essence where there is a chronic lack of vitality and low energy state, also for convalescence and never–well–since situations. It has a sluggishness and slow metabolism very much like the *Calcarea–carbonica* picture.

Peach Flowered Tea Tree has a strong affinity with the metabolism, digestion and the regulation of blood sugar levels. It's very helpful when there are hypoglycemic tendencies with resulting energy and mood swings.

Macrocarpa is useful for adrenal exhaustion, a classic burn–out picture. For someone who has been living on caffeine for too long, having too many late nights, working too many long hours, having much in common with the homeopathic *Nux–vomica* picture.

Black–Eyed–Susan is useful for those who are caught up in the rat race, always on the go and exhausting themselves.

Tall Yellow Top supports those who feel alienated, disconnected, somehow separate from everyone else and not belonging.

Sunshine Wattle brings a lightness to those who are caught up in the struggle and strife of life and are unable to see anything positive in the future.

Bailey Flower Essences

Marsh Thistle is for those who are stuck in routine situations and they have a fear of change and of new things. This fear causes us to cling to that which is familiar, even if it is slowly killing us.

Sea Campion is useful for those who suffered early or traumatic separation from the mother and feel insecure as a result.

Bach Flower Essences
Hornbeam and Olive are useful for a loss of strength and vitality, a feeling that they do not have the resources to cope with daily affairs.

Aspen and *Mimulus* help to alleviate the fears and anxieties that can drain our vital energies over time.

Lightbringer Essences
Aragonite supports us in feeling safe and secure in the physical body that we inhabit.

Hawthorn Blossom helps us to remember the abundance that we have in our lives when we get caught up in focussing on the lack.

Grandmother Pine helps us to reconnect with the ancestral wisdom that we carry deep within our psyche, reminding us of our dependence upon the great mother earth at times when we might feel shaky and unsafe.

Sycosis
Growth & Reproduction

I am fairly sure that psora, sycosis and syphilis are a trio in and of their own right. Psora is the pivotal point, the backdrop, upon which everything else depends. We cannot live on the earth and not be subject to survival issues, and we share this first challenge with the animal kingdom and every other living organism.

With psora as the pivot point, I started looking at sycosis and syphilis as complementary opposites. When I did that, I found them much easier to understand. I realized that in many respects, syphilis is everything that sycosis isn't, so they complement and oppose one another. This is helpful, because when you learn one of them, you already know the other, as a mirror–image.

In homeopathy, sycosis has to do with overproduction, discharges, heart disease, sexual disease, and a tendency to excess. There is too much catarrh, and an excess of warts, growths, tumors, together with urinary and sexual problems.

Looked at energetically, sycosis is an expansive energy. It's an energy of birth, growth, abundance and proliferation, none of which are bad. In fact, there wouldn't be any life without them. We're talking about the process of life itself. Every living organism has the tendency not only to grow, but also to reproduce, and so there is an immediate affinity with the reproductive organs.

Growth occurs on many different levels, however, and we can explore how the sycotic influence affects us in different ways during different stages of life.

The Sycotic Challenges

Reproduction/Survival of the Species

When we reach the age at which we can reproduce, we find the irresistible impulse to do so, whether we like it or not, which ensures the survival of the species. While psora carries the blueprint for our individual survival, sycosis is concerned with the survival of the species as a whole, therefore it has a relationship to desire, sexual behaviour and reproduction.

This impulse to reproduce and thereby to perpetuate the species is, just like the survial instinct, common to all living things. It just so happens that the sexual organs are among the most sensitive areas of the human body, which creates the possibility of sexual activity being both exquisitely pleasurable or intensely painful depending on the consciousness that we bring to it. In human life, sycosis includes the realm of sensuality as well as sexuality.

The countless social, religious and cultural taboos that have been imposed on the natural sexual impulse has given rise to all manner of sexual health problems, which the sycotic group of remedies are able to address. Prominent among these would be *Medorrhinum, Thuja, Staphysagria, Pulsatilla, Natrum– muriaticum* and *Sepia*.

Another related phenomena that the sycotic energy represents in neutral terms is the power of attraction. Positive and negative poles, masculine and feminine energies being attracted to each other happens throughout the animal and plant kingdoms. I would equate that with the sycotic miasm—the attraction of opposites with a view to creation, giving birth to something entirely new.

The Water Element

Psora seems to have a primary relationship with the earth, but we know that life on earth depends on water. Sycosis, then, represent our relationship to water and the watery element. We know that our physical bodies are at least seventy percent water. Many of our bodily functions involve the movement of fluids, whether it be urine, bile, blood, sexual fluids, mucous discharges or perspiration.

The sycotic influence keeps the fluids moving in the body, and promotes an adequate balance of the right fluids in the right place at the right time. In a healthy state, we drink when we're thirsty, empty the bladder when we need to, and by this means we neither retain too much water nor do we become dehydrated. The capacity to absorb, utilize and eliminate fluids is one of the physiological aspects of the sycotic influence. Energetically, this relates to the second or sacral chakra, which has a primary affinity with the genito–urinary organs and the gonads.

Boundaries

The sycotic miasm has to do with boundaries between the self and the rest of the universe. It's a semi–permeable energy boundary. We have to be able to allow certain things in and project certain things out and yet remain healthy. We can get sick from being too open, and taking in too many impressions. Conversely, if we shut ourselves down and don't allow anything in, we lose touch with our feeling function and this will create suffering also.

The sycotic is much more to do with the sensual, feeling side of life, whereas the psoric has to do with what is safe and secure. They overlap in this respect. When we reach a certain level of discomfort, we turn on the heat or the air conditioning to restore the feeling of comfort. Sycosis allows us to go beyond comfort and survival needs towards the enjoyment of what is desirable and pleasurable for us. It extends our sensory faculties into all kinds of areas such as the enjoyment of food, drink, sexuality, touch, music and dance. However, we have to know where to draw the line between what is good for us and what is not, and this is a big part of the sycotic challenge.

Sexuality/Sensitivity

Developing the feeling–sense and refining our emotional sensitivity is another aspect of the sycotic challenge. In order to deepen our relationships beyond the purely sexual level we have to learn to relate on an emotional level also, and this leaves us vulnerable to being hurt emotionally.

Finding a healthy balance in the area of sexual desire and fulfilment is also part of this miasmatic challenge, and it is by no means guaranteed that such a balance can be achieved. Sexual abuse in its various forms often leaves an imprint of emotional and psychological wounding, and many people are crippled with sexual guilt, shame or self-disgust as a result of early childhood experiences or conditioning. *Thuja, Staphysagria* and *Lac-caninum* are leading remedies in these states.

In some cases, the sexual energy can become obsessive or out of control, and we find indications for remedies such as *Hyosyamus, Platina* and *Medorrhinum*. In other cases, we find the sexual energy is blocked as a result of earlier traumatic experiences, or perhaps from hormonal imbalance as is seen in the picture of *Sepia*. How we relate sexually is a good indicator of how we relate to ourselves in terms of body–image and self–esteem, as well as revealing much about our emotional development and sensitivity towards others.

In *Medorrhinum*, on the one hand, there is a person who is so acutely sensitive that someone merely touching their hair can drive them into a frenzy. It's unbearable. Or, that person might look at a tree and burst into tears with the beauty of it. It's completely overwhelming, a whole–body experience of inter–connectedness with nature, animals or people. That's one side of *Medorrhinum*.

The other side can be a person who is cruel and hard–hearted, to their children or their pet dog or cat, for example. Someone who is outwardly cold, hard and cruel is often inwardly very sensitive. Either they were not allowed to be that way because they were judged for being 'soft' or 'weak', or they found it too painful to be that open and vulnerable, so they shut themselves down completely and lost touch with that inner sensitivity. The remedy *Anacardium* would be another example of this.

In order to be open energetically, we have to know that we are safe and are not going to be ridiculed, abused or harmed in some way. Even though we may be with a caring and loving partner now, the cellular memories of earlier traumas remain active within us, and nowhere is this more acutely felt than in the sexual realm. Healing these wounds so that we can enjoy healthy and fulfilling sexual relationships is part of what the sycotic miasm requires us to do.

Mental & Emotional Aspects of Sycosis

Growth/Expansion
Part of the sycotic challenge has to do with growth, not only on the physical level but also psychological and emotional growth, an expansion of consciousness. This, I believe, is pre–programmed into the genetic code of humans. Together with meeting our survival needs and satisfying our reproductive urges, we have an inbuilt need to expand and grow inwardly. We need to take on new concepts, ideas and possibilities, and we have to allow our self–identity to outgrow earlier forms and expand into new ones.

Ego Development
Sycosis gives us the first hint that we were never separate. If I can feel someone's presence without seeing, hearing or touching them, I am already awakening to the fact that we're connected. The message of sycosis is that we are all connected energetically, and as a result we can empathise with another. That is one of the gifts of sycosis, and many of the sycotic remedies have that in common.

I feel that sycosis has to do with the development of the ego, which means creating a sense of being an individual self, the notion that *this is who I am*. And again we have a paradox. Sycosis demonstrates to us how interconnected we are by our energetic links, and yet it also provides us with the internal sense of being a separate individual 'self'. We create a dialogue in our head about who we are, which we call 'ego'. Ego is actually a self–creation. Egotism or self–importance is a theme in sycosis, and is especially strong in *Medorrhinum* and *Cannabis–indica*. First we create a self, and then we gratify it with endless ego–driven desires.

Desire
If psora takes care of our needs, sycosis takes care of our wants and desires. Psora is very much concerned with essential

survival needs, what we need to stay alive and healthy. Sycosis allows us the comfort and luxury to go beyond that and say, *'Now what would I like? What gives me pleasure?'* Only when your basic survival needs are taken care of are you free to explore your preferences and to enjoy the wonderful sensual and sexual side of your nature.

Desire in itself is no problem. It's that we become attached to the object of our desire, so that we must have it. And when we have it, the satisfaction is only momentary. We only get temporary gratification and then we want it again, or we want more of it.

We are born with the innate tendency to have desires. It is desire that attracts things toward us. We magnetize experiences, people and possessions into our life because of our desires. It's not a bad thing. The question is: what do we really desire, what do we want to bring into our lives, and what do we do with it, having brought it there?

Space/Time
On the earth plane, we humans are required to function in a space-time reality. Events have a past, a present and a future. Things seem to happen sequentially, and we establish cause–and–effect relationships based on that linear sequence. Nature operates not in straight lines but in cycles, yet there is still a natural sequence in which things occur. If a person has problems with time and space in their life, think of the sycotic miasm. You can't have a problem with one without the other, so closely are they interlinked.

Having a problem with time is very popular these days. Many people are in a constant hurry. If you study the sycotic nosode *Medorrhinum*, these people are always in a hurry, constantly rushing from one thing to the next. That is an aspect of the sycotic influence that we haven't adapted to very well in modern society, giving rise to the sense that there's not enough

35

time in the day, or that time is passing by too quickly.

Sycosis can also distort our time–sense in the opposite way. In *Cannabis–indica*, a leading sycotic remedy, a minute can pass, and it seems like hours. It feels as though time passes incredibly slowly, and the person has all the time in the world. All of the major hallucinogens can distort our perception of time.

The psoric influence has to do with the seasons and cycles of nature, which are governed outside of us according to the movements of the planets. We have to align ourselves to nature's cycles in order to stay healthy. That's what psora is all about. Sycosis is about our own *internal perception* of time, and how we perceive time determines how we experience it. Time can seem to expand or contract depending on the situation we're in, and how we relate to that situation. It's either a gift or a curse. The gift is we can make time our own. The curse is that we feel we don't have enough, or that we have too much.

Once when Einstein was asked to explain his theory of relativity, he said that half an hour in the presence of a beautiful girl seems like just a brief moment, whereas a moment sitting on a hot stove seems like half an hour! So we can have an internal experience of time that is completely at odds with clock–time, and this can feel good or bad according to the situation we're in.

Memory
The sycotic remedies can have a great deal of trouble with memory, which is another facet of our relationship to time. *Medorrhinum* is the classic example, losing the thread of a conversation and forgetting what they were talking about. Hunting for specific words is a major *Thuja* symptom. *Nux–moschata* puts the laundry in the fridge and the milk in the washing machine, that kind of absent–minded forgetfulness and poor attention span. All these are manifestations of the fact that our perception of time has become distorted.

There has always been an association between marijuana and sycosis in homeopathy, and *Cannabis–indica* and *Cannabis–sativa* are listed as leading anti–sycotic remedies. Apart from the genito–urinary affinity, there is often a history of marijuana and other hallucinogenic abuse when the sycotic influence is dominant. What does marijuana do for us as a drug? It distorts time, expands consciousness, and changes our perception of space also.

Relating these phenomena to the chakras, I would say that the sycotic miasm has a primary affinity with the brow and the sacral chakras together. In my practice I have often see an imbalance in these two chakras in the same person. The brow chakra has to do with an expansion of consciousness, opening the third eye and expanding the inner vision. The very impulse to expand our consciousness is a sycotic drive. One of the ways we can do that is by ingesting psychotropic substances, hence the relationship between marijuana and sycosis.

Clairvoyance
The sycotic miasm seems to be concerned with perception through the energy body as a whole. The idea that perception is limited to the brain and the five senses is a relatively recent, western viewpoint. Ancient cultures held the view that we perceive with our whole energy body. You know from your own experience that you can feel somebody else's presence in the room. The scientist Rupert Sheldrake has conducted experiments with the feeling of knowing when someone is watching you, even when you can't see them. Somehow, you can feel their energy body impinging on yours, and his research has demonstrated that this is a very real and demonstrable phenomenon.

Energy body interactions as well as the ability to sense energy and to extend our energy outwards is part of the sycotic miasm. I would therefore associate the clairvoyant group of remedies with this miasm also.

Passion to Compassion

One of the challenges of this miasm is to take the passion, the sexual energy, the raw animal urge to reproduce, and to transform it into compassion. We have to take the energy from the sacral chakra up to the heart chakra, so that we can connect not only sexually but also emotionally, at the heart level.

In my opinion, ecstasy (also known as MDMA) is such a popular drug these days because it seems to open the heart centre. It is classified as an *empathogen*, which means it induces a temporary state of empathy and open intimacy. The problem is that there is a built–in tendency to repeat the drug and to want more, because after you've experienced it, ordinary relating and ordinary sexual relations can seem shallow and empty by comparison. The chemical itself is not considered to be addictive, but the feeling–state that it induces certainly can be, because we are longing to feel that deep heart–connection with our fellow human beings.

The fact that heart disease is the biggest single killer in the western world suggests that we are struggling with this challenge to relate to each other at the heart level. Meat consumption is also a factor in this equation, not only because of the saturated fats. In order to eat meat, we have to suppress our compassion for animals to some degree. Only by being open–hearted can we respond genuinely to other humans also. When the heart is closed, we tend to respond from a cold, intellectual and rational place, which means shutting off that part of us which feels and empathizes.

Global Aspects of Sycosis

If the miasms apply individually, they must apply collectively and if they apply collectively, they could also apply globally. If we look at some of the global issues we are now facing, we have massive economic expansion and population growth. As a direct consequence of economic expansion, we have global warming. Already we can see some sycotic themes emerging.

By burning up the fossil fuels, it seems that we are heating up the planet and releasing excessive amounts of carbon dioxide into the atmosphere. As a result, the fluids which are the lifeblood of the earth have begun to be affected. Ice sheets are melting, sea levels are rising, droughts and floods are both on the increase.

We humans tend to make linear predictions, but nature operates in cycles and always seeks to harmonize. Wherever you have expansion and growth, a point is reached which is called maximum expansion, and then contraction begins to take place.

The hottest topic among astronomers is the 'big bang' of creation. They have already discovered how the universe was born out of a terrific explosive event some thirteen and a half billion years ago. First, they found that the universe is continuously expanding and evolving. That would be the energy we call sycosis.

Now the scientists have discovered 'dark matter,' the limits to continuous expansion, and there is serious consideration being given to the 'big crunch', the antithesis of the big bang. We can surmise that eventually will come the great contraction, with global cooling, most probably another ice age. Where there has been a proliferation of life and growth, decay and death naturally follow. Syphilis and sycosis are equal and opposite influences. They balance and complement each other, just like yin and yang.

If we create more life artificially, it seems that nature creates more death. The spring and summer seasons are the sycotic, that which gives birth, growth, reproduction, expansion. Then we have maturity, followed by decay, contraction, decomposition, breakdown and death, which equates to what homeopaths call the syphilitic miasm. And this of course is the autumn and winter time, when everything returns to the earth. It is dark and cold and is associated with the night.

All of the major syphilitic remedies have their aggravation time in the winter, the cold, the night. Sycotic remedies are typically worse in the day–time, from heat, damp, during spring and summer. Conception occurs in nature during the quiet time, and gestation is at first hidden and protected. In the spring, we see the green shoots of new life emerging once again.

James Lovelock's Gaia hypothesis views the earth as a living organism. This viewpoint was shared by indigenous people the world over. Mother earth is subject to the same cycles and influences as we are. The forces of growth, birth and expansion, followed by contraction, decay and death happen on a cellular level, for individual plants, animals and people, for the whole earth, and now the physicists say, for the whole universe. The operating principles are the same, only the scale is different.

Addressing the Sycotic Challenge

The sycotic miasm is associated with the physiological imperative to keep fluids moving around the body in a healthy way. Wherever the bodily fluids become stagnant or hardened, the sycotic remedies are likely to be needed. A tendency to form kidney stones or gall stones, growths, tumours and swellings or deposits in the joints are typical sycotic ailments.

Fluids accumulating or stagnating locally in the body can give rise to ailments such as humid asthma, sinus congestion or oedema. *Natrum–sulphuricum* would be a leading remedy for asthma due to an accumulation of phlegm, and you will also see *Pulsatilla, Kali–Sulphuricum, Medorrhinum, Natrum–muriaticum* and *Thuja* frequently indicated for these watery sycotic ailments.

Consider *Medorrhinum* also for puffy ankles or feet, and for people who wake up with swollen fingers or wrists. When there's a sudden, big, fluid–filled swelling of the knee, *Medorrhinum* is one of the best remedies to get the fluids moving again. *Ruta–graveolens, Rhus–toxicodendron* and *Bryonia* may help a little, and then you look at the bigger picture, and you will see a sycotic tendency there.

To summarize, the sycotic miasm seems to have to do with birth, growth, reproduction, fertility and attraction—not only sexual attraction but any kind of desire, that energy which attracts things toward us. This relates to the ability to manifest and materialize, to bring things into our lives. The sycotic miasm also governs all of our sensory pleasures, our wants in addition to our needs.

Also, there is this awakening sensitivity, the capacity to feel energy with our own energy body and to notice how it interacts with other energy fields. Finally, the sycotic also relates to an expansion of consciousness, which often leads to or includes some kind of psychic development or expanded perception.

Each of these qualities that the sycotic miasm represents can be considered neutral in essence, which means they will have both a positive and negative pole. The negative side of desire is when it turns into greed, the desire which is never satisfied. The negative side of sexual attraction could be lust, promiscuity or an addiction to sex or pornography.

The negative side of expanding consciousness could be someone who feels a connection to the whole cosmos, but who is too spaced out to make breakfast. If you are too 'out there', the everyday things can seem unimportant and get neglected, so we have to find a way to stay grounded while we expand.

The negative side of developing sensitivity is that it can be so painful that you feel you have to shut down or protect yourself and then a shell of hardness or even cruelty can develop. The negative side of abundance is that we think that there's a limitless supply of everything. Because nature is so abundant, we think that we can take more than we need without regard for the long term consequences. We can easily confuse abundance with excess.

A lot of people suffer with sycotic ailments these days. Heart disease we've already mentioned, which relates to closing down the heart centre. A lot of heart disease is due to a clogging of the arteries, which is primarily a dietary issue. Yet what we eat, how that food is produced, and how much we eat are all a reflection of our current state of consciousness. You can't really separate the two.

There is a fast growing grassroots movement towards sustainable agriculture, organic produce and compassion in the treatment of farm animals, and I would see this as positive evidence that we are collectively beginning to wake up to the sycotic challenge.

My current understanding is that the sycotic and the syphilitic entirely complement one another. Sycosis and syphilis go together because they're two ends of the same pole, whereas psora stands alone, as a midpoint between them. The end of the cycle of expansion and growth is the beginning of the cycle of contraction and death. At that changeover point, we move into the syphilitic energy. They flow into each other, just as the seasons flow into each other. It's a process rather than an event, and you will see different miasmatic influences take precedence at different stages in a person's life. As one miasmatic influence wanes, another one becomes activated.

You can see that process most vividly in children who are undergoing homeopathic treatment. You can give a child *Medorrhinum*, and a month later, they come back with clear indications for *Tuberculinum*, and you may wonder where that came from. They come back again, presenting indications for *Syphilinum* and you might think, '*should I be giving one nosode after another*'? Yet that is what they seem to need. And that's the nature of these miasmatic energies, that they all blend, one into the other, with no fixed boundary between them.

If we see any of the key sycotic themes showing up in a person's life, or manifesting as symptoms and health issues, we can support them in developing a harmonious relationship with this energetic influence. Depending on the individual, we may need to encourage an opening of the heart or reconnecting with the sensuous side of their nature. For someone else, the challenge may be to expand their consciousness and to allow their psychic sensitivity to open up, if it is ready to do so.

Some people may need help with grounding themselves and finding a way to connect with their earthly roots, and this is essential for those whose psychic sensitivity is opening up. I have often recommended gardening, manual activities or some kind of bodywork for people who have a tendency to become spacy, unfocused and disconnected as their consciousness expands. If you want to have your head in the clouds, you need to find a way to keep your feet planted firmly on the ground.

Flower Essences for the Sycotic Miasm

Australian Bush Flower Essences
Fringed Violet is indicated when the auric field has been damaged or traumatized through any kind of abuse, violence, injury, drug use or shock. It helps to heal and repair the energy bodies and reduces any over–sensitivity to environmental influences.

Consider this essence for people who are too open energetically and they take on everyone else's impressions. They feel things too acutely, so it's painful for them. They pick up on other people's feelings, vibrations, energies, or even diseases. They can walk under a power line and get a headache. It is a useful complement to remedies such as *Phosphorus* and *Medorrhinum*.

She Oak as its name implies, has an affinity with the female hormones and reproductive organs and helps to regulate any imbalance in this area.

Wisteria and *Flannel Flower* are very useful essences for sexual blocks such as frigidity or painful sex, particularly where there has been a history of sexual abuse. Also indicated where there is a fear of intimacy or sensuality.

Sundew helps those who are dreamy and tend to drift off to stay grounded and focused in the present moment.

Bailey Flower Essences
Thrift is for those who are developing their intuitive or psychic abilities, and they need help staying grounded while developing their inner vision and psychic sensitivity. It helps a person to open up gradually, especially where they may have become frightened by a sudden expanded perception in the past, such as can happen after drug use.

Bracken (Aqueous) helps those whose psychic sensitivity was blocked in childhood, with a resulting fear and mistrust of the intuitive faculty.

Welsh Poppy is for those who are unfocused, ungrounded and spacy. It is helpful for grounding, keeping a person connected to the earth and preventing them from spacing out.

Hairy Sedge helps with memory problems, where the person can remember many things perfectly but certain things are impossible for them to remember. Sometimes specific memories have been rendered inaccesible because they are too distressing or painful to recollect.

Tufted Vetch is indicated where there is a confusion of sexual identity, sometimes with a history of sexual abuse.

Algerian Iris is useful where the sexual energy is overly dominant and the person is driven by a desire for sex into unsuitable relationships.

Bach flower essences
Clematis, like the *Welsh Poppy* is useful for people who are ungrounded, spacy or unable to focus. It is a useful complement for remedies such as *Opium* or *Medorrhinum*.

Walnut is useful for protecting against outside influences and also helps with breaking addictions and negative habits.

Lightbringer Essences
Bogbean helps a person to find the balance between over–sensitivity on the one hand and insensitivity on the other. It helps those who are over-sensitive to find the optimum degree of sensivity without becoming hardened and closed.

Pink Purslane supports a deepening experience of a person's sexual and sensual nature on all levels. It encourages a gentle opening to deeper levels of sexual intimacy and trust, and is useful where there is a history of sexual wounding or abuse.

Venus Transit helps with opening to the energy of the divine feminine within, balancing the male and female aspects for both men and women.

Vernal Equinox has a cleansing and clearing effect on the sacral chakra, awakening and releasing the sexual energy where it has been obstructed.

Syphilis
Death and Destruction

The syphilitic miasm represents the forces of decay, breakdown, contraction, destruction and death, none of which are inherently bad. It just happens that we have a cultural prejudice against them, and we have a selective bias in favor of accumulation, birth, growth and expansion.

In modern western society, economic expansion is considered a 'good thing'—we are encouraged to want bigger houses, more goods and more money. If we were a healthy society, we would have an equal relationship with growth and decay, expansion and contraction, life and death, with no discrimination.

The syphilitic influence, as a neutral force, teaches us not to get attached to the things that we've created and accumulated, because everything in nature is transient and changes form sooner or later. We suffer when the things we have become attached to are taken away from us, which everything is, eventually. This is one of the core tenets of Buddhism, to recognize the impermanence of the outer forms of life.

While the sycotic force pushes outwards and is ever–expanding, the skeleton, flesh and bones draw the boundary for us in our physical bodies. The strongest affinity of the syphilitic miasm is with the bones and skeleton, the physical structure, which gives a certain order to and defines the limits of the body–mind. If we expand our consciousness yet neglect the limitations and requirements of the physical body, we will suffer.

One of the wonderful paradoxes of life is that it would be impossible to sustain life on this planet, were it not for the process of death. If we weren't breaking down cells at the same rate that we are producing them, we would die from the over–production of cells. The equilibrium between the forces of life and death is how we maintain health, and the same is true of all life–forms on planet earth.

The Syphilitic Challenges

Inner Darkness

On the psychological level, I feel that the syphilitic miasm represents all the things associated with the winter and the dark, which is a time for turning inwards. If the sycotic miasm expands our consciousness, our perceptions, our exploration of other dimensions and other worlds, the syphilitic represents the *inner world* and forces us to go inside, into our own hidden depths.

The syphilitic miasm has always been associated with darkness and the night. The syphilitic anxieties, depressions and most of the pains of the syphilitic remedies are aggravated in the dark, during the winter and at night.

Culturally, we have a prejudice against the dark, the winter and the night, and we try to mitigate its influence upon us. We keep the lights on and the fires burning, not only from survival necessity, but also to prevent us from getting too close to our own darkness. In psychological terms, the syphilitic has to do with the shadow aspects of ourselves that we don't want to look at.

It is the equivalent of the 'dark matter' and 'black holes' that the astronomers have discovered in the outer reaches of our universe. We have within us the deep, dark ocean of the unconscious realm. One of the roles of the syphilitic miasm is to remind us that we also have to turn inwards and to recognize our own depths. We have to do as much inner work as outer work in order to grow and develop as healthy human beings.

Interestingly, most of us venture into the inner world only when we are forced to by life, when everything we have built up suddenly gets stripped away. It is usually a death or a collapse, a business failure or marriage breakdown, the kind of events we associate with remedies like *Aurum–metallicum*, that

50

causes us to question our life values and to turn inwards. Most of it is forced upon us. If we visited this place voluntarily more often, the involuntary encounters with our shadow side might not need to be so frightening.

We create problems for ourselves by avoiding the darkness completely, or by going in there and losing our way. There's a potential for great despair and a spiraling down into hopelessness. You see the deepest, darkest pits of depression and despair among the syphilitic remedies such as *Aurum, Syphilinum* and *Mercurius*. All of the demons that frighten us the most exist inside of us. Nothing in the outside world compares to the things that we can encounter in our own psyches.

One of the Bailey flower essences, *Moss,* is indicated for a fear of the shadow side. *'Fear of the dark spaces within'* is how Arthur Bailey describes it. This essence is helpful when you know that there is something there, you can't quite see it but you feel this thing stalking you and lurking in the background. It can manifest in the form of panic attacks or nightmares and you don't know where they come from, there is just a sudden, overwhelming fear.

The things 'out there' are only a reflection of what is inside you. In fact, the perspective of several spiritual traditions is that everything we see manifesting outwardly is a projection of our own mind. It's a collective hallucination. If we were to change the internal consensus, the outward appearance also changes.

Think about how we learn what things are. We teach children the consensus of what a chair is, its functions and form. If we didn't teach them that, we have no idea how it would appear to them. We know that when photographs were first shown to Native Americans, they only saw an amorphous, blurry image, because they had no existing reference point about what a photograph was. When you break down your conditioning, your world literally begins to collapse, and this is the main reason we cling strongly to the collective values.

One way we attempt to deal with the darkness inside is by shutting it out with drugs, alcohol, or workaholism. We block the awareness of it and distract ourselves by various means. These self–destructive behaviour patterns are all strongly associated with the syphilitic miasm.

We can also develop a very distorted image of ourselves. We can create monsters where they don't exist. We can see ourselves as being horrible, dirty, disgusting, loathsome, and it's all a fabrication of the mind, often the result of negative childhood conditioning. This is also a syphilitic tendency seen in remedies such as *Lac–caninum, Syphilinum* and *Mercurius*.

Egocide
The syphilitic miasm seems to break down the structures that are no longer needed so that new ones can replace them, and this includes our ideas of who we are. The sycotic miasm builds up an image, an idea of who we are, known as the persona. There comes a point where we begin to realize that this isn't who we are at all, it was just a self–identity that we adopted for a while.

Often we get attached to our roles in life, and we identify ourselves with them. The destructive syphilitic force comes along to remind us that's not who we are at all by stripping it away and showing us that we still exist. Therefore, that can't be who we are. It was just an illusion, albeit a very persistent one.

For example, I used to think that I was a homeopath. Some of you reading this book probably still think that you are a homeopath. When you immerse yourself in something as fully as many of us do with a topic like homeopathy, it actually becomes who you are for a time. It's an identity–structure that, once created, becomes part of the self–image.

But there comes a time when what you've created no longer serves you and instead becomes a limitation, and that's the point where the syphilitic energy awakens. It's a boundary that has become too tight, too restricting. To my own surprise, homeopathy became a straightjacket for me, and calling myself a homeopath didn't feel entirely true any more. I was still using homeopathy some of the time, but I could no longer identify exclusively with being a homeopath and I began to let go of my attachment to that role. It is not an easy process, especially when you have invested a lot of time, energy and money in becoming that which you say you are.

There is this important aspect of the syphilitic that has to do with ego death and letting go of the idea of who we thought we were. It seems to be happening to an enormous number of people. All of the existing forms and structures and roles that people have been quite comfortable in for hundreds of years no longer work. Many people are losing their jobs, their relationships and other forms of outer security.

If you look around you will find a lot of people going through either a relationship or career trauma, a mid–life crisis or some kind of existential breakdown. If, as healers, we are going to be of service to those who are undergoing these necessary life transformations, then we need to have some awareness of the process and we have to engage and work with it within ourselves.

Breaking Down/Letting Go
The breaking down of old forms and structures brings a lot of chaos into people's lives. I can only presume that we need that chaos, that it serves to show us where we were becoming too attached to the outer forms of life, and to the false images of ourself also.That these structures get demolished is not inherently bad, but of course it can be painful, especially if we cling on through fear.

One of the main spiritual teachings is non–attachment, not to get too attached to our creations and the things that are given to us. Everything in life is given on loan. When it's taken away, it feels like we have lost a crucial part of ourselves, something we can't live without. And of course, we didn't.

One of the lessons of the syphilitic tendency is the lesson of letting go. The degree to which we can continuously and repeatedly let go, preferably consciously, is the degree to which we don't have to suffer with syphilitic illnesses or syphilitic behaviors. The destruction we associate with the syphilitic miasm is often just a stripping away of something we have been clinging to that in fact we no longer need.

Control/Chaos
One of the polarities of the syphilitc miasm is the balance between control and chaos. When someone is struggling with the syphilitic tendency, there is often the feeling that they are on the verge of losing control. You can observe that it takes an increasing amount of will power for this person to keep it together, to prevent their life as they have known it from falling apart. This suggests that the person is grappling with the emerging syphilitic energy inside.

Mercurius, Arsenicum–album and *Aurum–metallicum* try to keep things stable and under control on the outside, but they feel increasingly unstable inside, and not much is needed to push them over the edge. The tendency towards ritualistic and obsessive behavior is also syphilitic. Consider the obsessive remedies like *Argentum–nitricum*. This is a way of trying to impose some order on a seemingly chaotic universe. The person will think, *'Perhaps if I count every single railing along the street, I'll be all right.'* That could be one way of keeping it together on the way to the office.

One of the biggest fears that arises during a time of personal transformation is the fear of insanity, of losing control of the mind. That fear can be expressed in countless ways in the course of a consultation. I would say it is one of the deepest fears that people are collectively feeling now. What isn't necessarily realized is that the old structures *need* to be broken down, let go of or even destroyed.

The normal response to that fear is to hold on to the familiar, to cling to the old structure even more tightly. This is the *Arsenicum* dilemma. You will often see this remedy picture arising when a person is getting close to death, and they are clinging to life by the fingernails. The decay and death of the body is the ultimate loss of control, and the ego knows it.

Purification

Traditionally, purification has always been associated with fire, and I would associate the fire element with the syphilitic miasm. Fire is a symbol of destruction and breakdown, but also of transformation. Nothing is entirely consumed through fire—it gets purified and transformed into something finer. The ash, which is the refined essence of what came before, always remains.

If you want to create a nice pot which is going to last, it has to be fired. That is how it gets its strength. This is one of the great alchemy teachings—the base material has to go into the crucible. And psychologically speaking, so do we, and not just once! Fire always brings gifts that we would not be able to access any other way, but we have to be able to handle this volatile energy and find a way to contain it while it does its work of purification.

Some years ago, I heard the Irish homeopath Nuala Eising give a talk about her proving of *Fire*. Somehow she captured fire and turned it into a remedy and conducted a proving, and she took it herself, as well. She demonstrated in the conference how she had prepared the remedy and almost burned the conference hall down in the process, which was interesting in itself.

While the provers were taking the *Fire* remedy, they felt an uncontrollable impulse to clear all the clutter out of their lives. The provers would go home and look at their house and say, *'This place stinks. That's got to go, that's got to go.'* They became completely ruthless. Nuala went through her house and got rid of all the curtains, half of the furniture and most of the cats. Everything had to go, and she had this compulsion to paint the walls white.

Everything had to be clean and purified. And that's the energy of fire taken to an extreme, which is what a proving is. It's an exaggerated form of an energy that many of us need in our lives now, the energy of clearing out the clutter, emptying ourselves voluntarily and stripping away that which is no longer needed.

If you ever hire a feng shui consultant to take a look at your living space, one of the things you can be certain of is that they will tell you to clear out all of your clutter. When we accumulate and store away things that we no longer need and, in many cases, don't even like, we are obstructing the natural flow of life energy and storing up trouble for ourselves. Sooner or later, that stagnant energy will find a way to start moving again.

Addressing the Syphilitic Miasm

In the Thomas gospel, one of the gnostic texts found in Egypt in 1945, there is a quote attributed to Jesus which says: *'If you bring forth what is within you, what you bring forth will save you. If you do not bring forth what is within you, what you do not bring forth will destroy you.'* To me, that has to be referring to the psychological shadow, an aspect of the unconscious psyche, and I feel it reflects the issues of the syphilitic miasm very accurately. If you make it conscious and work with it, it will save you. It will be exactly what you need to develop and to grow in your life. If you deny it and push it into the unconscious, it will leap out and grab you, always when you least expect it.

Meister Eckhart, a thirteenth century German mystic, said, *'The soul grows by subtraction, not by addition.'* If you look back on a period of psychological or spiritual growth, you'll generally find that it's when you've let go of something that you have made progress. It's the letting go that allows you to expand and grow. These are the lessons of the syphilitic—surrender, letting go, allowing things to break down in their own time and even encouraging them to do so when necessary. If you perceive that the time is ready for something to break down, then do it willingly. If you work with it, rather than against it, you can prevent a lot of suffering.

One of the manifestations of *'what you do not bring forth will destroy you'* could be a person who suddenly has a big accident. We associate the syphilitic miasm with accidents, but where do accidents come from? One school of thought says there are no accidents, that we create them. We don't create them consciously of course, but we could well be doing so unconsciously. Carl Jung was of the opinion that whatever we deny and push into the unconscious will tend to show up in our life as some kind of fateful event.

Accidents, sudden illnesses and other traumatic events can be viewed as wake-up calls from the unconscious to tell us we need to change direction. If a person works with that, it can be a transformational period in their life. I've seen a number of business people who were totally driven, workaholic types and suddenly they've had an accident, and having spent weeks and weeks in bed, they are forced to look inside. It can be harsh medicine if we don't listen to it, address it, and work consciously with it. We have to give it emphasis now, because our social and cultural tendency is to deny the dark, to ignore the shadow and the unconscious realm. We have to be willing to look at what is there and bring it into the light.

Another teaching to be found in many spiritual traditions is that you have to be emptied before you can be filled. I remember Arthur Bailey telling me a story from the zen buddhist tradition. A man was seeking guidance from his spiritual teacher. He was relating all of his problems, talking non–stop. The spiritual teacher sat there absolutely calm and quiet. Then he said, *"Would you like some tea?"* The teacher poured the tea until it was overflowing, and when the man protested, the teacher said, *"That's just what you're like. Your cup's too full already. There's no room."* We have to be emptied before we can be filled. Most of us get emptied involuntarily.

Embracing Death

Elizabeth Kubler–Ross did a great deal of work raising the consciousness around the processes of death, dying and letting go. In recent years, a whole mass of literature has been published about the near–death experience. Many thousands of people who have clinically 'died' under anesthetic, from a heart attack or a major injury, have survived and returned to tell the tale. This is breaking down our outmoded ideas of what it means to die.

Generally, in western culture, we have come to view death as a finality, an end, and consequently death has become something to be feared and avoided. Medical science has become obsessed with the prolongation of life at all costs, and it is considered to be a failure of medicine when a person dies.

Many of the people who have died and resurrected tell a remarkably similar story. Usually they experience going down a dark tunnel, into the darkness, and then they see the light at the end. The darkness is always followed by an opening into the light, and frequently they are met by the smiling faces of relatives and friends, or they find themselves feeling completely safe and secure, as if all their fears and insecurities had been erased.

Thousands of people have reported a similar experience, independently of each other, of going into the darkness and then experiencing the light and the expansive opening into something quite glorious. It is such a graphic image, and it's striking how closeley the death process mirrors the birth process.

In the sufi tradition they have a saying: *'Die before you die'*. The idea is to let your false–self die away while you are still alive. Indeed, this is the most powerful way to really come alive and to live life in its fullest expression of your divine origin. A research study was carried out on the individuals who had jumped from the Golden Gate bridge in San Francisco with the clear intention of ending their life, but had nonetheless survived the ordeal. It was found that they had all been transformed by the experience in a positive way, 'coming back to life' as it were with a renewed spirit.

Many ancient cultures understood the necessity to die before you die, and created elaborate death–and–rebirth rituals to carry the initiate through from one stage of consciousness to the next.

Most of us have neither the resources nor the support that would allow us to take a month or two off work or take a sabbatical to fall apart when we need to. We don't have the cultural support for that either. Consequently, we may have to fall apart in little stages, while we're still looking after the family, holding down a job and paying the bills. This is where the help and support of a practitioner can make all the difference.

Right now, we are going through a collective transformation of consciousness. As practitioners, I believe we need to extend our repertoire beyond simply using remedies to cure diseases. We can include flower essences and other tools to support the transformation process, and we can cultivate relationships of equality and trust with our clients to help them in ways that do not encourage dependency on the practitioner.

On a global scale, I would equate the syphilitic energy with that which inevitably follows a sycotic period of great expansion, population growth and global warming. What follows is a period of global cooling, the next ice age, a great contraction and ultimately, the 'big crunch'. This would be the syphilitic energy, translated to the universal level. I don't know how many tens of thousands of years these cycles take but it seems that we are getting closer to some kind of tipping point.

Summary
As I understand it, the major challenge of the syphilitic miasm is to allow to die that which needs to die, when it needs to die. To embrace death in equal measure as we embrace life, and to practice non–attachment. Another part of this challenge is to draw appropriate boundaries and to create appropriate structures for as long as they are needed, without making them too fixed or too rigid. Just as our physical body needs both a physical structure as well as flexibility to function, the structures we create also need that same flexibility.

Another aspect of the syphilitic is to be willing to go into the inner dark spaces, and not be deterred by our fears of those places. We need to cultivate a willingness to go into the unconscious realm regularly and voluntarily, without always waiting until it comes knocking. There are many routes to the unconscious, including the exploration of dreams, via the arts, or through astrology and other forms of divination.

When Carl Jung was introduced to the Chinese oracle known as the *I-Ching*, he was initially skeptical of its value. Experimenting with it soon caused him to change his mind, however, as he found it to be an uncanny mirror of his own unconscious process. His theory of synchronicity was formulated as a result of these researches and parallel discoveries that were being made in the field of physics.

Flower Essences for the Syphilitic Miasm

Australian Bush Flower Essences
Grey Spider Flower is particularly helpful for intense, phobic–type fears and nightmares. It can help those who feel they are under some kind of psychic attack.

Waratah is for the 'dark night of the soul' stage, where a person needs to summon all their strength and courage to stay with their inner process and not give up in despair.

Dog Rose of the Wild Forces is for the fear of losing control, when the emotions are overwhelming and too intense.

Mint Bush is for those who are going through a 'spiritual emergency' of some kind and are struggling to maintain their balance.

Bailey Flower Essences
The whole group of Bailey essences are related to personal transformation, offering support through the different stages of self–growth. They are particularly helpful when a person feels stuck and is unable or afraid to move forward.

Leopard's Bane is indicated for the feeling of being on a knife edge, where a person feels that they could lose it at any minute. When someone is exercising a great deal of control, often the fear they have is that an impulse will arise that will be harmful to themselves or others. This is also the *Mercurius* dilemma, the feeling of an impulse to do harm, to do violence, and it frightens them.

Moss helps with the fear arising out of the unconscious that something is lurking in the depths that will jump out and grab you.

Bistort helps to build a kind of 'inner scaffolding', which is needed during periods of internal transformation. When your life is falling apart in some way, and you know it needs to, and you're working with it as best you can but feeling insecure and vulnerable at the same time, **Bistort** helps you to keep on track and gives you that feeling of much–needed inner strength. It helps a person to keep their faith and to trust that they will make it through a difficult period.

Yew is for those who refuse to bend, who get rigidly fixed in one place or with one idea or attitude. Despite the fact that life is coming at them like a steam train, they refuse to budge. In tai chi, the more rigidly you stand, the easier you are to push over. True strength comes from flexibility, which gives you the ability to yield to, absorb or evade a strong force that is coming towards you. The lesson of *Yew* as a flower essence is to stay supple and fluid, to keep moving, to go with the flow and to bend with the forces that come towards you rather than to rigidly resist them.

Blackthorn is useful for anyone who is struggling with deep depression and despair, who perhaps is being treated with homeopathic *Aurum–metallicum* or *Syphilinum*. This is described as the black pit where there is no light, no hope, a feeling of utter hopelessness. There are two flower essences that are similar in that respect. The other is *Gorse* from the Bach essence set. I would say that **Blackthorn** is a more severe depression.

These are both shrubs that flower in the winter. When everything else is asleep and apparently dead, both *Gorse* and *Blackthorn* come out in full bloom, bringing the solar light of consciousness exactly at the time when it is most needed.

Bach Flower Essences
Cherry Plum is for those who are almost cracking under the strain and are afraid of breaking down completely, losing

control of the mind or acting on dangerous impulses.

Crab Apple helps with the feeling of being unclean in some way, which relates to the *Syphilinum* compulsion to be always washing their hands.

Gorse is for hopeless despair, very similar to the **Blackthorn** already mentioned above.

Sweet Chestnut supports those who are at the very edge of breaking down with despair or depression, they may feel that there is nothing left to live for.

Lightbringer Essences

Fly Orchid helps to embrace and make friends with our inner darkness so that we can transform it into something positive and life–enriching.

Ruby in the Storm supports a person in staying centred and grounded while in the very midst of a major life upheaval. It helps them to go with the flow and surrender to the necessary change, despite the fear and confusion that may arise.

Silver Birch helps with harnessing the inner fire energy in a positive rather than a destructive way, burning away false illusions and protecting against the abuse of this potent energy.

Tuberculosis
The Divine Wake-Up Call

This miasm could be called the light at the end of the tunnel. While the whole of nature continues to give birth, expand, contract and then die, it seems that we humans are given other options. One of those options is what we have come to associate with the tubercular miasmatic influence.

There is a moment of readiness when we can transform that circle into a spiral. Out of the emptying process can come new hope, inspiration and creativity. This is not just a return to an earlier state, but a breakthrough to a whole new level of consciousness. Many of the best creative works arise out of the ashes of depression, despair or great hardship. When a person goes through the darkness and finds their way to the light, they often emerge with a new insight or a different awareness of some kind.

I would equate human aspiration, spiritual awareness and creative potential with the tubercular miasm. It allows humans the possibility to break out of the purely animal, instinctual, material realm. Within us also is the desire to explore and experience things outside the cycle of death and rebirth, which takes us into other realms. *Aspiration* is an interesting word. On the one hand, it means a desire to improve things in your life, to have a worthy goal or ambition that you are *aspiring* towards, but the same term also refers to the act of drawing substances into the air passages.

Many spiritual traditions emphasize the importance of the breath, and a central idea is that the life energy itself is carried through the breath. Breathing is one of the few bodily processes that we can consciously influence and exercise some control over. We can hold the breath, deepen it, speed it up or slow it down. We can utilize the breath for self transformation, and we can engage with our own body via the breath. This equates to the air element, which has to do with travel, communication, creativity, art, music, painting, dance and an appreciation of nature and of beauty.

The Tubercular Challenges

Dissatisfaction

Another word that expresses this relationship between the breath and our inner life is *inspiration*. The things that inspire us I would equate with the tubercular. Why does the *Tuberulinum* individual feel restless and dissatisfied? Why are some people satisfied with what they've got, and others are not?

The tubercular type has a sense that things could be changed or improved, or that there is something missing. There's a part of them that isn't satisfied by any of the everyday activities, any of the ordinary things that they've pursued up until now. This person may have succeeded at work, or in raising a family, and they have achieved what they set out to achieve in life, but there is a feeling of '*and yet....*' That feeling is the seed of potential that we equate with the tubercular miasm. It is the feeling that *there must be something else to life, some deeper meaning....* and of course, there is!

This is the seed that drives us to re–ignite the memory of our connection to the divine realm from which we came. I feel that the tubercular miasm is related to that divine seed which is planted within us. It has been called '*the urge to merge'*, and it is said to be something which lies dormant in each of us. It is like a little seed, a time bomb, which ticks and ticks and when it finally goes off, it takes that person on a whole new path.

Something has been awakened that nothing this person has done until now will satisfy. They will try everything to satisfy it. This is what we call the *Tuberculinum* pathology. They will travel to the corners of the earth, hoping to find it, whatever it is. They don't even know what it is, but they hope to find it. It's a fire in the heart. It may lead them into music or art, sex or spirituality, poetry or romantic love. Tuberculosis used to be called *consumption*, and not without good reason. This fire is an all–consuming desire and passion. It comes from a different place. Neither sex nor food will satisfy it. *Tuberculinum* types can eat as much as they like, and they won't gain any weight. Traveling won't satisfy it. They feel that the grass is always greener somewhere else.

Homesickness

Where do you really find the answer to this eternal longing? When, like the prodigal son, you finally come back home. And the only place you can really be at home is inside yourself. One of the main psychological states associated with the tubercular trait is *homesickness*. Sometimes we feel homesick when we get displaced from where we grew up, or when we are exiled from our homeland, but there's another level of homesickness that has nothing to do with location. It's an internal homesickness. You could call it a homesickness for the divine, for a connection with your true self. It's something we look for outside that can only be found inside. The end of the journey is back at the beginning. Yet we come back changed, potentially at least. If we come back before we're ready, we may have to take the journey again until we are truly satisfied.

Freedom

Once the tubercular seed has taken root, there will be a drive for freedom, and a resistance to any kind of restriction. You'll see this in tubercular children. If you put a tubercular child on your lap and wrap your arms around them, they'll break free. They hate being restricted. If you put a tight sweater on them, they'll feel like they are suffocating. As they get older, the things that restrict them will start to feel more and more oppressive. At one age, it's a sweater, and at the next age, it's living with their parents, and then it's being in school, and then it's living in England. There are levels to it. Breaking through those freedom barriers is one of the driving forces of the tubercular.

A desire to escape is another part of the pathology of the tubercular remedies. An example would be the remedy *Iodum*, the ultimate tubercular remedy. It has the fastest metabolism, they can eat and eat and eat, and yet lose weight. This is a hyperthyroid picture, and they hate being restricted in any way. They want to escape or run away, and in the extreme state if you oppose or restrict them, they can become violent and even murderous.

Violence

What lies just behind the tubercular miasm is the syphilitic. If you see someone in the tubercular phase and you try to squash them, it brings out the syphilitic, the destructive element. They will either destroy you, or themselves, or both. That is why I think *Tuberculinum* and *Syphilinum* are mutually complementary remedies. If someone does very well on one of these, very often they will need the other. If you think that *Tuberculinum* should help and it doesn't, it is worth trying *Syphilinum*. Often it seems that we need to complete the syphilitic phase before we can progress fully to the tubercular.

If you suppress the tubercular urge, it will tend to bring out violence towards others or some kind of self–destruction. The tubercular person cannot be thwarted and stay healthy. It is like a point of no return—there's no going back from being tubercular! You can go through this stage and move on and take it with you. But you cannot go back to being an 'ordinary' person living an ordinary life. You may try this for a while, but ultimately it will not satisfy.

Heaven and Earth

One of the big tubercular challenges is balancing the routine with the sublime. On the one hand, we still have to pay the bills and take care of our responsibilities and, at the same time, a part of us knows that there is something more important in life than any of these things. We may have only the vaguest notion of what it is, and yet we have an urge to seek it. This can feel like being pulled in two directions at the same time. One of the hardest challenges is how to reconcile ordinary family

69

or work life with the spiritual or creative life. Jack Cornfield's excellent book *After the Ecstasy, The Laundry* addresses exactly this dilemma.

Many of the spiritual traditions have tried to overcome this paradox, often by advocating renunciation of worldly things such as sexual relationships or possessions. In the sufi tradition, they take a more practical approach and encourage the followers to lead a normal family and work life, so that the sycotic impulses and desires will not be a source of distraction from the spiritual path. The idea is to be *'in the world, but not of the world'*, which is far from easy.

Lungs/Breath

The tubercular miasm has always been associated with the breath and with lung problems. The most favourable place for a tubercular person is said to be up in the high mountains. This is the air element of course, but it also has to do with aspiration. When we aspire towards something, we instinctively tend to seek a high place. It's no coincidence that so many spiritual retreats and monasteries are built on mountain slopes. It helps to get a different perspective from up there.

Problems with restrictive breathing or constriction around the throat are almost always reflective of someone who is struggling with self–expression in some way. Often it is simply that the person needs to reconnect with their creativity. There may be a creative spark that has been dampened down. Typically, a person who used to sing or paint or write poetry got caught in the mundane aspects of raising a family or earning a living, and they forgot whatever it was that used to inspire them.

When the tubercular influence is activated, the creative impulse gets reawakened, and if you don't listen, it will start to consume you, one way or another. Often it manifests symptomatically in the chest and throat area, or in the thyroid gland. You will often see thyroid problems and throat problems in general, in people who have been thwarted in terms of their own self–expression.

There is a strong relationship between the sacral chakra and the throat chakra. The sacral is called the *lower creative*. It governs sexual attraction leading to procreation. The throat is called the *higher creative*. This takes us beyond the purely biological, instinctual level. The impulse here is to create as an expression of our connectedness to the divine and mystical realm. When the throat centre is opened, there is a potential to create something uniquely beautiful, inspiring and uplifting. The most sublime creative works arise not from a place of pain, but through the direct expression of divine energies which can only flow unimpeded when the channel is open.

A useful practice for people having problems in this area is to wear a piece of turquoise or a turquoise scarf around the neck. Turquoise as a gemstone or even just the colour will strengthen this area and help the throat centre to open.

A number of homeopathic remedies display the dual affinity for the sacral area and the throat. *Folliculinum* is considered to be helpful for suppressed creativity, particularly where a hormonal imbalance is part of the picture. *Lac–caninum* is another remedy targeting both the genitalia and the throat. *Lachesis* is the same. With *Lachesis*, there is an excess of sexual energy which gives rise to the loquacity for which the remedy is famous.

Heart/Romance
The great sufi mystic Rumi wrote that *'Remembrance makes people desire the journey. It makes them into travelers.'* What is the remembrance of which he speaks? This is the remembrance of our true spiritual nature, which gives rise to this longing to be reunited with our source.

Another driving force of the tubercular miasm, related to the heart connection, is the urge to merge with a partner, not just on a sexual level but on a heart level. This connects to what was mentioned earlier about the use of ecstasy and the opening of the heart centre. Many young people today know intuitively that they have to connect not just sexually, but from heart to heart and on a spiritual level also.

A cultural obsession of the western world, which we are happily exporting to the rest of the planet, is romantic love. Since the time of the troubadours, romantic love has been held as the highest ideal of love, as it has all of the qualities of a divine visitation. Very often, the heartbreak that is suffered in the name of love is but the painful cracking of the shell that precedes a breakthrough to a greater level of awareness. Romantic love, which is a very personal form of love, can be a gateway to the greater, impersonal form which is the divine love.

The homeopathic remedies that relate to romantic love have a relationship to the tubercular miasm. When we fall in love with an ideal rather than a real person, disappointment is the inevitable consequence. *Ignatia* and *Natrum–muriaticum* are the leading remedies for this tendency, and *Luna* also.

Calcarea–phosphoricum, Phosphorus and the *Ferrum* group are also strong tubercular remedies. The *Ferrums* have to do with oxygenation and the blood supply. Flushing and flushes of heat are also tubercular indications on the physical level. Wherever oxygen or the air element is disturbed, think of the tubercular miasm. It could be hot flushes with sweats, or they can feel very chilly and yet are easily overheated.

Displacement/Imprisonment
Tuberculosis as a disease is associated with two main phenomena—being displaced from one's homeland and being forcibly trapped or imprisoned against one's wishes. The disease often takes hold among refugee and immigrant populations, in prisons and encampments where people are forcibly kept, or

in any conditions of severe overcrowding. In Britain there has been a high incidence of tuberculosis among Asian and Indian immigrant populations who have often been forced to live in overcrowded conditions.

Losing one's sense of home or what home is awakens the tubercular. The challenge of the miasm is to learn that *home is where the heart is* — ultimately, it is to be found inside us, and we can feel at home wherever we are. A great many people are on the move during these challenging times, and it is no surprise that the incidence of tuberculosis is rising in many regions. We are still grappling with the tubercular challenge, and the great spiritual awakening which has been predicted is very much a work in progress.

Hope/Idealism

Balancing hope with idealism, creativity and boredom, everyday activities and inspirational acts is at the heart of the tubercular dilemma. The tubercular energy is a restless energy, and if it is not harnessed carefully it can lead to an endless cycle of disappointment and unrealized ideals.

Every growth in consciousness comes at a price, and the tubercular is no exception. While the longing for something meaningful can bring forth a passion for life and a drive to experience the full mystery of being human, it can also bring a great sense of frustration and emptiness as the struggles of everyday existence begin to lose the value they once had.

Restriction/Freedom

Another polarity is restriction versus freedom. One of the lessons of the tubercular is that true freedom is never found by running away or escaping. No matter how far we may travel on the spiritual quest, we are always heading in the same direction—back home to ourselves. *The kingdom of heaven is within you*, Jesus said. We know this intuitively, but it doesn't prevent us from searching far and wide.

Ultimately, real freedom is found within yourself, but travel can certainly catalyze the process and speed it up. When we cross cultural boundaries, our conditioning gets challenged on a daily basis and we are forced to give up a little part of who we think we are. We get so used to our cultural values that we don't even know they are only part of our conditioning, not part of being human.

I only started to notice these things when I began to travel. Traveling can be a necessary catalyst for inner growth. It's very difficult to break down your cultural conditioning while you remain in the culture in which you grew up, just as it's very difficult to access your family patterns and beliefs if you never break free from your family. We have to balance travel versus escape, and be alert to that restless desire for a change of scene that takes us nowhere.

The tubercular miasm equates to the planet *Mercury*. It also has elements of the sun, with the heart affinity. But especially it relates to *Mercury*, the traveler, the messenger, the communicator who brings the messages of the gods to the people. That is the essence of the tubercular challenge—finding a way to integrate the creative, spiritual life into the acts of daily life.

Flower Essences for the Tubercular Miasm

Australian Bush Flower Essences
Bush Fuschia is a wonderful essence for opening the throat chakra and assisting with self–expression and creativity.

Boronia is for those who are pining or longing following a broken relationship. It helps to heal a broken heart.

Silver Princess is for those who have lost their direction and are drifting, feeling flat and lifeless and in need of inspiration.

Sturt Desert Pea helps to release deep hurt, grief and sadness from the heart area.

Turkey Bush is for blocked creativity, writer's block and such like, or to help a person connect with their creative side.

Bailey Flower Essences
Lily of the Valley is for people who feel a constant yearning or longing for something beyond and greater than what they have. This longing is a key feature of the tubercular urge to reconnect with one's source.

Pine Cones is for someone who feels trapped or dominated by another person's authority. They feel squashed and thwarted and unable to lead their own life.

Scarlet Pimpernel is a complementary essence for those who are unable to free themselves from another's influence. Even though they may be physically separate, still they may be trapped by the psychic or energetic bonds which connect humans who have been in intimate relationship with each other.

Oxalis is indicated for the feeling that someone or something has you by the throat and they are holding you there, refusing to let you break free. The person will often develop throat problems with no actual throat pathology.

Bach Flower Essences
Honeysuckle helps a person who is prone to nostalgia or homesickness, who is longing for life to return to how it used to be at some earlier time and place.

Wild Oat helps a person to get 'on track' with their life, when there are numerous possibilities but no clear direction. This essence was instrumental in aligning me with the path of healing and homeopathy at a time when I could easily have been distracted by other pursuits.

Lightbringer Essences
Alpine Forget-me-Not supports the remembrance and the experience of divine love as a true presence in one's life and not just as a concept.

La Meije relates to the 'divine wake-up call' and helps a person to go beyond their own limits and take the necessary leap of faith into the unknown.

Cancer
Self in Relationship to Others

It's very difficult to think of the cancer miasm in neutral terms, because the word 'cancer' has so many negative connotations. Just hearing the word affects your energy body. It triggers images and associations in the psyche. It is so ingrained in us to be afraid of cancer as a disease, that it's hard to think of the miasm as a neutral energetic influence. However, I did attempt to approach the miasm in this way, and I began by thinking of the well-known remedies that have the strongest affinity with the cancer miasm—remedies such as *Carcinosin, Staphysagria, Thuja* and *Natrum–muriaticum.*

I realized first of all that the cancer miasm has a great deal to do with relationships between human beings. Interestingly enough, cancer as a disease rarely affects the animal or plant kingdoms, except when humans are involved. Domesticated animals frequently develop cancer, but it is relatively uncommon amongst wild species in their natural habitat.

I feel that both the tubercular and cancer miasms are challenges that are specific to humanity, whereas the psoric, sycotic and syphilitic influences affect all life forms on planet earth. The tubercular and cancer miasms, and perhaps some of the newer miasms now being considered seem to be the optional extras that we humans take on board.

The very prevalence of the various forms of cancer despite the massive efforts of modern medicine to 'make it go away' suggests that this particular miasmatic challenge is being grappled with collectively on a major scale. I was astonished in my homeopathic practice at how frequently *Carcinosin* seemed to be needed by people of all age groups, and I found this was true not only in the U.K but in most other countries that I have visited also.

The Cancer Miasm Challenges

Personal Relationships

Socially and culturally, we are being forced to address our relationships now and to recognize the significant role they play in our psychological and emotional growth. Virtually everyone faces some kind of relationship challenge in their life, whether it is with a partner or with family members, friends or work colleagues. Ram Dass called relationships *'the yoga of the west'*, recognizing that this is where we do most of our growing, albeit unconsciously much of the time. If you want to run a busy healing practice, I would suggest making a study of relationship issues and see what you have to offer in that area.

With the tubercular miasm, the urge is to experience something in the hope that it will fill the spiritual void that is being felt. We are seeking an experience—be it mystical, romantic, artistic or creative—which will transcend the ordinary and provide a taste of the extraordinary. With the cancer miasm, we are being pushed to experience something specifically *in relationship to our fellow human beings*. The cancer challenge is concerned with developing our innate human qualities of compassion, love, empathy and individual self–identity. I would say that this miasm is primarily concerned with our individual, one–to–one relationships.

One part of this challenge would be how to stay open emotionally and yet feel protected and safe at the same time. How can we be kind and caring towards others but not so naïve that we get abused and trampled on and end up feeling like a victim? This side of the cancer miasm challenge can lead to the *Staphysagria* pathology, of being too accommodating and agreeable, to one's own detriment. *'Whatever you say, dear, is fine with me.'* The doormat syndrome. Underneath the submissive facade is seething anger, because of the continuous suppression of a part of the self.

A variation on this theme is taking on someone else's whole way of being, such that we identify with it and begin to think that's who we are. This happens when we allow someone to dominate us because we feel subservient and secondary to them in some way, or we believe they know better than we do. Gradually we begin to lose our sense of 'self', and this, I believe, is the key to understanding both the cancer miasm and the nosode *Carcinosin*.

Individuation

A major theme that is relevant to the cancer miasm is the journey towards individuation. Carl Jung coined the term *'individuation'* to describe the process of becoming a whole human being, a whole person in your own right, and living your own life to its fullest expression. He said that we often look for, in other people, that which we sense we are lacking within ourselves, or which lies dormant within us and we haven't yet been able to access, develop and express. We tend to seek that in a partner, and also in our role models, in the people we admire, and we must learn to discern what is truly ours and what belongs to someone else.

The process of becoming whole is inextricably linked with engaging with other people, because we try to become whole by attracting people towards us who have the very qualities that we are unconsciously seeking to develop within ourselves. This is a difficult challenge, because we can easily get stuck in a state of co–dependence if we are not careful. A co–dependent relationship is one in which we believe that we cannot be complete or function fully without having a certain person in our life.

A further challenge here is how to become a whole person in one's own right and yet not become closed and isolated. This is the *Natrum–muriaticum* side of the cancer miasm. *'That person hurt me, so I am going to be independent from now on. I'm not going to rely on anyone but myself.'* Closing down emotionally is a natural reaction when we have been wounded, but sooner or later we must find the courage to open our heart and learn how to trust again.

A related remedy which also addresses the theme of individuality is *Lac–humanum*. The challenge with this remedy is the conflict between pleasing oneself versus pleasing the family and conforming to their expectations and demands.

Suppression/Conformity

We know that suppression is a major issue in the cancer miasm. We see it especially in the remedies *Staphysagria, Thuja* and *Carcinosin*. It's not just emotional suppression, although that is a major component. I would say in more general terms that it is suppression of one's individuality, in whatever way that manifests. It has to do with being something that you're not, or being *someone* that you're not. I think more than anything else, this is what tends to activate the disease side of the cancer miasm.

We compromise ourselves sometimes to fit in with another person. I've seen that so often with people who have active cancer. I've had clients consult me with an early–stage localized cancer who are firm believers in alternative healing, and who are otherwise in good health. There is absolutely no reason why they couldn't have at least a reasonable chance of recovery through natural treatment. I would ask, *'What are you going to do?'* And the client would answer, *'Chemotherapy and surgery. My husband would worry if I didn't.'*

That's the essence of the cancer miasm dilemma—going against your own sense of what is right for you, even if it might kill you. *'He'd worry if I didn't have the chemotherapy. I wouldn't want to upset him. And the doctor was really nice.'* That kind of attitude which is so prevalent in British culture is undoubtedly a contributory factor in activating the disease aspect of the cancer miasm. The tendency to try to please others, to go along with other people's opinions and not to upset anyone, can be deeply ingrained. Research amongst cancer sufferers has shown that the 'difficult' patients who question everything and refuse to do as they are told tend to have better recovery and survival rates than the 'good' patients who are more docile and compliant.

There is also a scenario where one partner has cancer for many months or even years, who subsequently dies, and then their partner who was nursing them also develops cancer. They have become over–identified with the role of being a carer for the other person. It's as if their entire life's purpose became limited to being a care–giver. Again, that's the over–sympathetic aspect. When the caretaking role gets taken away, they can feel as if there's nothing else to live for.

Edward Bach, the flower essence pioneer, warned against this tendency in his little booklet *Heal Thyself*, and developed a group of essences around the theme of *'Over–concern for the welfare of others.'* Bach had a malignant tumour removed from his spleen at age thirty-one and subsequently died from cancer at the age of fifty, so I would presume that he was writing from his own experience.

On a wider scale, the pressure to conform can be seen as part of the challenge to our self–identity, and this is a particularly powerful influence if it operates at a societal level as well as within the family and peer groups. As we progress through adolescence, there is a healthy throwing–off of the authority and expectations of those around us which is essential if we are to find our true individual path in life. In some cultures, the collective pressure to conform is overwhelming and the needs of the individual are always subsumed under the demands of the group.

When you consider the kind of repression that is applied under totalitarian regimes, this I would see as the same challenge being played out on a larger scale. With communism, for example, part of the ideal was to erase the differences between people and thereby create a kind of pseudo–equality. In Europe, we have seen how the ideal of a European Economic Community has in many cases proven to be detrimental to the interests of individual groups. If we have learned anything from our experiments in large–scale industrialized agriculture, it ought to be the recognition that *nature favours diversity over conformity.*

Self–Esteem

There's another aspect to the cancer miasm tendency that I call *'false humility.'* It is part of a lot of religious conditioning of the kind that tells you to hang your head low, to accept how miserable and guilty you are, and then you'll be okay. This attitude doesn't do much for healthy self–esteem or healthy relationships. On the contrary, it makes for abusive relationships. If we put ourselves down and abuse ourselves, we invite others to treat us in a similar way. If we raise our self–esteem and learn to take care of and respect ourselves, we engender respect from other people. We unconsciously invite abuse into our lives when our attitude and behaviors demonstrate that it's okay for us to be treated this way.

Many people are taught that if they look after themselves and put themselves first, they are being selfish. They learn to associate taking care of their own needs with feeling guilty, and compensate for this by putting everyone else's needs and wishes before their own. Over time, resentment inevitably builds up and the person loses touch with what their own desires and needs really are. Developing healthy self–esteem and self–respect are part of the cancer miasm challenge.

This is the axis on which *Carcinosin* and the cancer miasm rest, on relationships and self–esteem. You cannot separate those two. If someone works on improving their damaged self–esteem, all of their relationships will change. And if someone wants to improve their relationships, they usually have to work on developing their self–esteem. They are inseparable.

Taking Responsibility
The cancer miasm is also about taking responsibility. If we don't take responsibility for our lives, we tend to fall into a pattern of blaming someone else or blaming ourselves, and developing a victim mentality. Ultimately, the cancer miasm teaches us to be responsible for our own life choices and to be true to ourselves.

I believe that when we are true to ourselves, this doesn't generally lead to selfish behaviour. On the contrary, we can offer the best support to others only when it comes from a place of genuine compassion and open–heartedness, and not from a sense of duty, obligation or being over–sympathetic. This is very different from helping others from a place of being wounded ourselves, and needing to help others as a distraction from our own suffering, which is the unconscious tendency of the wounded healer.

Self-Identity
Carcinosin is the only nosode that didn't have its own proving. The picture of *Carcinosin* was developed by Donald Foubister, relatively recently, in the 1960's. Foubister studied several hundred women who were pre–cancerous or post–cancerous. He looked at the patterns, tendencies and emotional states of these women and drew a picture of the remedy. This picture was subsequently expanded through the clinical experience of many homeopaths. *Carcinosin* is a collection of lots of different individuals. It doesn't have its own identity, and this is the *Carcinosin* problem.

The *Carcinosin* type typically has a poor sense of self–identity. There is a lack of certainty about who they are as an individual, and because of that lack of certainty, they have a tendency to adopt other peoples' attitudes, beliefs and behaviours.

Carcinosin, when you first study it, looks like every other remedy all mixed together. It has keynotes of *Lycopodium, Pulsatilla, Thuja, Natrum–muriaticum, Nux–vomica, Arsencium–album* and *Staphysagria,* among others. That is actually one of the indications of *Carcinosin,* when two or three or four polycrest remedies all seem equally well–indicated.

The *Carcinosin* tendency is to identify with and then take on other people's issues, and become something which is not true self. Often after a successful prescription of *Carcinosin,* the person will return with a clear picture of one remedy. They may come back angry and frustrated, a clear *Staphysagria* picture, or a clear, resentful *Natrum-muriaticum.*

This is a good sign, because it's genuine. *Carcinosin* strips away the false ways of being that were acquired and didn't really belong to the person, and reveals the true feelings that were underneath. Not everybody is happy with this outcome, of course, and I've had clients complain to me that they were unable to keep up their appearance of being nice to everyone after taking the remedy.

Cancer - The Disease

Cancer as a disease seems to accurately reflect many of the themes being discussed here, particularly with regard to the boundaries between self and other. When cells become 'cancerous', they either begin to replicate uncontrollably in one locality, and/or they start to invade neighbouring tissues and may even metastasize to a different location altogether.

The common theme here is one of aggressive self–assertion of an individual group of cells, with an apparent disregard for the well–being of its neighbours and relatives. It seems as if the cancerous cells are displaying exactly the kind of self–centred behaviour that the person themselves would find unacceptable, albeit to an extreme degree.

When someone develops cancer, they are often forced to break an habitual lifelong tendency to put everyone else's needs before their own. Perhaps for the first time in their life, they have to assert their own needs and wishes. They may have to stop taking care of others and allow themselves to be taken care of.

Cancer also brings the difficult challenge of standing up for oneself and differentiating between what does and doesn't belong to you, what is good for you and what is not. Making treatment decisions based on what your own heart tells you rather than blindly following what the 'experts' and the people around you are saying can be incredibly difficult, yet absolutely necessary, for someone who has active cancer.

Having observed many people struggle with the reality of cancer in its various forms, I have come to the conclusion that the kind of treatment regime someone follows is probably not the single most influential factor in determining the outcome. I've met many people who have undergone orthodox treatment procedures and have lived to tell the tale, and just as many who have had every kind of alternative treatment yet still they didn't survive.

For me, the really crucial question is whether or not a person's consciousness has been transformed by the whole experience. If it has, I'd say the prognosis is always more favourable, irrespective of the type of treatment being followed. And if it hasn't, I would be much more alert to the possibility of relapse or recurrence of the disease, perhaps in a different form.

Homeopaths and the Cancer Miasm

Homeopaths and healers are certainly not immune to miasmatic influences. If anything, I'd say we are more susceptible than the general public, particularly when it comes to the cancer miasm. The nature of our work should tell us that we need to actively engage with these processes. If we are to have any hope of helping other people, we have to learn to help ourselves, and the fact remains that homeopaths do get sick and develop serious pathologies just like everyone else.

As healers we are in a position of vulnerability, and the cancer miasm is always there as a teacher. We have to know how to relate to our clients and be open and compassionate, but without identifying too closely with other people's problems. We must distinguish between what is ours and what belongs to the people we're working with. We have to maintain clear, healthy boundaries to prevent overwhelm and burn–out. And we have to avoid taking responsibility for other people's well–being and life choices.

Homeopaths are very good at examining other people's problems, analysing cases and 'curing the sick', which is very much in the Hahnemannian tradition. We have yet to fully recognize that we ourselves are the wounded healers who are struggling unconsciously with exactly the same issues we see reflected in our patients. I would say that self–growth, self–awareness, self–responsibility and self–healing need to be built into every healing profession. Only from that position can we really be of any help to anyone else.

Addressing the Cancer Miasm

The biggest affinity of *Carcinosin* is with the blood and the immune system. The immune response creates a semi–permeable barrier between oneself and the outside world, and between oneself and other people, in particular. Its function is to discriminate, to detect enemies and friends, allowing in that which is healthy, and keeping out that which is not. An important part of our immune response is the ability of the body to say *'no'*, and it is often exactly the same lesson that is being delivered by the cancer miasm.

Appropriate assertiveness in drawing one's personal boundaries is a key part of the cancer miasm challenge. We have to be able to relate openly to others and yet also be able to say, *'No, that's yours, and you can keep it, thank you.'*

When the cancer miasm is activated, very often the immune response is either over–active or under–functioning. This kind of imbalance reflects an issue with discrimination between what to let in and what to keep out. When a person is struggling with that issue, some things get let in that shouldn't be, and other things get shut out that actually need to be let in.

Multiple allergy syndrome is a physical pathology reflecting this issue, and *Carcinosin* is the main remedy for it. This is not just hay fever or milk allergy. It is an allergy to many different substances, all at the same time or constantly changing from one thing to the next. They are over–reactive to many different things, without the ability to discriminate between what is healthy and what is not.

When the cancer miasmatic tendency goes back all the way to childhood, there is often a history of severe or repeated childhood diseases or other infectious diseases, for example, getting the measles three times. For most of us, once is enough to develop healthy immunity. Or they have a history of sudden, recurring, high fevers of unknown origin, usually with swollen lymphatic glands. It's as if the immune response has gone into overdrive. The other extreme is a compromised immune system, an absence of immunity, often compounded by an excess of antibiotics and other suppressive medications.

Wounds that are slow to heal is also an indication for *Carcinosin*. There can be poor healing, poor recovery, poor convalescence and acute diseases that don't clear up. There are deep emotional wounds as well, from which the person has not been able to recover. Deep sadness, grief, guilt or anger, which is not helped by the usual remedies.

Another interesting clinical feature of *Carcinosin* is that it is the best remedy to help people recover from a blood transfusion, when they seem to be adversely affected by it. Again, this relates to the theme of self-identity which is so central to the cancer miasm. There is emerging evidence now from recipients of organ transplants suggesting that something of the 'energy' and even the personality of the organ donor gets taken on by the recipient.

Spleen Affinity

Another affinity of the miasm is with the spleen, which is very closely connected with the immune system. The spleen is often involved in cancer, particularly in leukemia, where it becomes enlarged. The spleen is an organ that is generally underestimated and misunderstood in Western medicine. It is regarded almost on the same level as the appendix, as some prehistoric leftover that we can well do without. Yet I've seen many people who have had their spleen removed surgically, and it is clear that they have lost something which is vital to good health.

In traditional Chinese medicine, the spleen is given equal status to the other major organs such as the liver, stomach and gall bladder. In this system, they relate the spleen to *sympathy*, which is very interesting when you think about *Carcinosin*, a leading remedy in the rubric *Sympathetic*. That means sympathetic as a pathology. To be overly sympathetic means identifying with someone else's problem and taking it on as your own. This person literally suffers when they see someone else suffering.

We have an expression in English called *venting your spleen*, which means expressing your anger and getting something off your chest. This is often exactly what a person displaying a *Carcinosin* picture needs to do, yet is unable to out of fear of upsetting someone.

Glandular fever, also known as mononucleosis involves the spleen and the immune system. The common name is the 'kissing disease,' and it is prevalent amongst youngsters in their mid to late teens. Kissing has to do with relationships, intimacy and boundaries, and relates directly to the cancer miasm. *Carcinosin* is the absolute number one remedy for a person who has never been well since glandular fever, even if they had the disease many years ago.

Summary
To me, the cancer miasm speaks of the need to go inside and reconnect with who you really are, which usually means letting go of what you thought you were. Often in the process of discovering who you are, you'll have to harness some of the destructive syphilitic energy and use it in a positive way. You may need to destroy some false ideas and get rid of the things in your life that are no longer serving you.

You may also need to grow and expand, and bring in some of the positive sycotic energy. If you have spent a lot of energy taking care of everyone else, you might have to uncover your own needs and desires and begin to follow them. You may also need to reconnect with your creative side. If you became a housewife or an accountant when you really wanted to be an artist, the tubercular creative urge may have been squashed within you. Just as the syphilitic fuels the tubercular, I would suggest that the tubercular fuels the cancer. You may see this in your treatment sequence. If a person responds well to *Carcinosin* and related remedies, you'll often see tubercular remedies appearing afterwards. Keep in mind that the cancer miasm embraces everything that precedes it, so that any of the other major nosodes may follow *Carcinosin* also.

The cancer and tubercular miasms might be seen as the transitional miasms. These are not just to do with cycles that keep going round and round until we break certain patterns. They are concerned with major life transformations, where a person is struggling to work through something internally and attempting to integrate a whole new level of consciousness.

Flower Essences for the Cancer Miasm

Australian Bush Flower Essences
Alpine Mint Bush supports healers and other care–givers who are in danger of burning themselves out through giving too much to everyone else.

Five Corners helps to raise self–esteem in those who have a poor self–image and a 'crushed' personality.

Monga Waratah helps a person break free from co–dependent relationships and to find their own inner strength.

Southern Cross is for those who are self–sacrificing, with a hidden resentment about feeling like a victim. It's a *'take pity on me, but don't help me'* kind of attitude, also known as martyr syndrome.

Bush Gardenia helps to renew the vitality in relationships that have become stale. A related essence, *Wedding Bush* helps with a fear of commitment in relationships.

Boab supports those who are attempting to break free from negative family patterns, which can sometimes run through many generations.

Bailey Flower Essences
Bog Asphodel is for the 'willing slave' who sacrifices their own needs while getting caught up in rescuing everyone else.

Butterbur is for those who are afraid to express their full potential as they believe it will have a negative effect on others.

Lilac helps those who have been dominated by others and whose growth has been hindered as a result. A related essence,

Pine Cones is for those who are still trapped by some authority figure from whom they are unable to break free.

Sumach is another Bailey essence that promotes healthy self–esteem, especially in those who refuse to accept their own potential.

Witch Hazel is for those who get stuck in a pattern of always trying to live up to other people's expectations, and they try desperately not to let anyone down.

Milk Thistle helps to open the heart chakra and to release the fears that hold a person back. It supports the gentle growth of self–love and self–acceptance.

Early Purple Orchid is a wonderful support essence for anyone who is transforming their self–image and developing healthy self–esteem.

Scarlet Pimpernel helps those who feel emotionally trapped by others to break free and to cut the hidden energy ties that can keep a pattern of dependency in place.

Bach Flower Essences

Centaury is for the 'doormat' mentality, the person who cannot say 'no' to others and struggles to assert themselves.

Cerato helps those who are unsure of themselves and tend to be easily swayed by other people's ideas and opinions.

Pine is for self–blame and self–reproach, guilt feelings and taking responsibility for other people's mistakes. This essence reminds me of the Englishman who says *'sorry'* when someone steps on *his* foot!

Red Chestnut is for those who are constantly worrying about other people and creating unnecessary anxiety for themselves.

Lightbringer Essences

Angel Star helps a person stay true to themselves and to their own voice during challenging times when confusion and uncertainty threaten to throw them off course.

Monkshood helps to develop a sense of what is 'good medicine' for each individual, illuminating what is both nurturing and also detrimental to one's well-being and vitality.

Primrose supports clarity in love relationships, helping to keep ones' personal boundaries intact while being open to the experience of loving relationships with others.

Chakras, Elements & Planetary Correlations

Once you have begun to relate to miasms as transformative agents, each one representing a certain type of energy, it is interesting to see how they overlap with other maps of consciousness that we are already familiar with. Three such maps that I have linked up with the major miasms are the seven–chakra system, the four elements and the seven–planet astrological system as described by Robin Murphy.

My own suggested correlations are given below. These things cannot be set in stone as there are always different interpretations and degrees of correspondence to be considered. Nonetheless, it provides a useful way of associating one kind of information with another. More detailed information on these topics can be found in my recorded seminars *Homeopathy and the Chakras* and *Health and the Planets*.

Psora
I would associate the psoric miasm with the base chakra primarily, and then the solar–plexus chakra. The corresponding element would be earth. The main planetary affinities would be Saturn (elimination, rectum); Jupiter (digestion, metabolism) and Mars (survival instinct).

Sycosis
The sycotic miasm seems most strongly associated with the sacral chakra and the corresponding element of water, and also the brow or third–eye chakra. The main planetary affinities would be Venus (genito-urinary organs, mucus membranes); Moon (fertility, hormones, fluids) and Jupiter (growth).

Syphilis
The syphilitic miasm I would associate with the fiery solar–plexus chakra as well as the base and heart chakras. The corresponding element would be fire. The related planets would be Saturn (bones, teeth, structure, decay) and Sun (heart,

despair). *Aurum–metallicum* (gold) is the metal that relates to the sun and is one of the leading syphilitic remedies.

Tuberculosis
The tubercular miasm has its strongest affinities with the heart and throat chakras, and relates to the element of air. Mercury (lungs, throat, communication) would be the leading planet, together with Sun (blood circulation).

Cancer
The cancer miasm as you would expect can be matched to almost everything, but I would say the strongest chakra affinities are the heart, solar–plexus and base. The Moon (cancer, lymphatics, breasts) would be the strongest planetary association, together with Venus (relationships), Jupiter (growth) and Saturn (death).

The Five Hindrances

In the Buddhist tradition, there are said to be five major hindrances to progress on the spiritual path, and these can also be aligned with the five major miasms.

The first hindrance is sensual desire, lust or greed, which clearly equates to the sycotic challenge. The second is anger, ill–will or aversion towards others, which I would associate with the syphilitic miasm. The third hindrance is sloth, torpor or apathy, which aligns with the psoric challenge. The fourth is restlessness, worry or dissatisfaction, which equates to the tubercular restlessness. And the fifth is self–doubt or lack of conviction, which matches the cancer challenge.

New Miasms

A number of new miasms have been suggested from a variety of sources in the last few decades. In the book *Flower Essences and Vibrational Healing* by Gurudas, it was suggested that there are a further three major environmental miasms for humanity to contend with, associated with radiation, petrochemical and heavy metal toxicity.

Amongst the homeopathic community there has also been speculation concerning an A.I.D.S. miasm, and other acquired miasms relating to diseases such as leprosy, ringworm and malaria. Of all these, the ones I have given serious consideration to have been A.I.D.S. and radiation. Radiation interested me mostly because I was living in Cumbria for thirteen years with a nuclear power plant on my doorstep that was famous for the frequency of its 'accidental' leaks of radioactive material into the atmosphere and the neighbouring Irish Sea.

As far as I am aware, the suggestions put forward by Gurudas have not been widely embraced, or even acknowledged by the homeopathic profession at large. This is unfortunate, and is probably due to the unusual source of the material as well as the esoteric nature of the text in which it appears. The Gurudas book, together with several companion volumes, were compiled from a huge volume of material obtained through the 'trance channel' Kevin Ryerson, who has worked as a professional psychic medium for many years in the tradition of Edgar Cayce. He became famous following the publication of Shirley MacLaine's book *Out on a Limb*, in which he featured.

By chance, I once mentioned my interest in miasms to a homeopath friend in California and he arranged for me to meet with Kevin Ryerson during one of my visits. After a brief introduction, Kevin offered to conduct an impromptu session for me so that I could ask any questions I had on the topic, and he promptly fell into a trance state. The first few words came from

'John', the spirit guide who oversees Kevin's work, and what followed was a surreal and yet completely 'normal' question and answer session between myself and 'Tom McPherson', a fifteenth century Irish alchemist who, apparently, was the expert on technical matters such as miasms.

When Kevin came out of trance at the end of the session, he had no idea what had been discussed, and was curious to hear anything I could tell him. While we had mostly discussed the well–known chronic miasms, which were the subject of my research at the time, 'Tom' had impressed me with his grasp of the subject and assured me I was on the right track in considering the miasms as related to stages of consciousness. Kevin, I would like to add, struck me as a genuine seeker for truth who was open–hearted and generous towards me, a complete stranger who turned up on his doorstep.

This meeting with Kevin Ryerson led me to take the idea of new miasms more seriously, and my subsequent studies of the Gurudas material opened up another dimension of this work for me. A key concept I discovered in the channelled material was the emphasis given to flower essences and other 'vibrational remedies' as well as homeopathy. It began to dawn on me that if we are to approach miasms from the viewpoint of consciousness transformation, then we will need to extend the repertoire of tools we use in our healing work, and 'Tom' seemed to be of the same opinion.

Flower essences, unlike homeopathy, were developed *specifically* to address states of consciousness rather than disease states, and as such I believe they are ideally suited to working with miasms in a more conscious and holistic way. Hence my decision to include some flower essence material in this book to illustrate how they can be used in practice.

A.I.D.S.
Self in Relationship to Society

I've had relatively little experience of treating patients with active A.I.D.S. and H.I.V.–related diseases, but have been interested to consider it from a homeopathic point of view. As with cancer and the other miasmatic diseases, it is hard to think of the A.I.D.S. miasm as something neutral with potential gifts as well as the destruction that it brings. There are, however, several themes that we can discern which suggest a miasmatic theme that is a direct continuation of the chronic miasms already discussed, particularly the cancer miasm.

When A.I.D.S. first began to be recognized, initially amongst homosexual males, it brought into consciousness a kind of plague mentality, with the corresponding attitude that those affected were contaminated and needed to be kept separate from the general population. The miasmatic challenge seemed at first to have to do with unconditional acceptance, as many of our collective societal prejudices and judgments were being brought to the surface by the spread of this so–called 'gay plague'. In this respect, we can see the kind of stigma that was previously associated with leprosy and the venereal diseases, especially syphilis, being activated once again.

Over time, it became clear that other sub–groups of the population were also susceptible to this new disease syndrome, most notably intravenous heroin users and haemophiliacs, suggesting that it was being transmitted somehow via the blood. There was, however, an undeniable element of sexual transmission being observed at the same time amongst other groups.

In sub-saharan Africa, meanwhile, the disease began to spread at an alarming rate amongst the general population, and was clearly being passed on directly to children born of infected mothers. Here, the risk factors seemed to be a combination of malnutrition and a weakened immune system due to other endemic diseases such as malaria and tuberculosis. Possibly the suppressive medications used to treat these diseases have played their part also.

How are we to make any miasmatic sense of this increasingly complex phenomenon? One thing we can deduce is that the A.I.D.S. miasm, if there is such a thing, is a hybrid of some if not all of the other chronic miasms. There is a clear relationship to the cancer miasm, with a shared immune–system and blood affinity.

Whereas the cancer miasm challenges us to clarify our sense of self in relation to other individuals, the A.I.D.S. miasm extends the challenge further to our relationship with society as a whole. This theme emerged in the proving of the A.I.D.S. nosode conducted by Misha Norland, where the feeling of being an outcast or not belonging to the group featured strongly.

The immune–system affinity suggests an association with boundaries, and another part of the A.I.D.S. miasm challenge may have to do with recognizing the limits of what the human body will tolerate. Whether the system breaks down due to drug abuse, malnutrition, promiscuity, repeated suppression of venereal and other infectious diseases or any combination of these factors, there has to be a point at which the body–mind declares: *'Enough is enough'*.

One of the lessons here may be a renewed respect for the body on every level, and also for the sanctity of human sexual relationships. On the one hand this miasm alerts us against making moral judgments and creating scapegoats, but on the other hand it seems to be showing us that we cannot treat the body as an object without suffering the consequences.

Radiation
The Responsibility of Power

If one of the lessons of A.I.D.S. is to remind us that there is a breaking point in the body, then radiation could be viewed as one of the breaking points of the whole planet. The cancer and A.I.D.S. miasms are very much to do with relationships between people, whereas the radiation miasm seems to go way beyond that. It is more global in its scope, and has to do with the power we humans yield and the ethical responsibility that power brings.

The application of nuclear radiation as an energy source as well as in bomb–making has shown us just how much power human beings can harness, not only for creativity but for destruction. We have come to realize that we have created the ability and the means to destroy the entire planet several times over. We have that as one of our choices. This shocking realization forces us to take responsibility, not only for ourselves, but collectively, on behalf of all humans and every other species also.

The technology that produced the atom bomb came from the research of physicists, and the writings of many of those same physicists are not unlike the writings of the mystics. They have, through their scientific research, established the interconnectedness of everything in the whole universe, thus confirming one of the ancient spiritual truths that was in danger of being obliterated from the Western psyche.

That to me is the wonderful paradox. The scientists have shown us how everything is connected to and dependent upon everything else, and they have also given us the potential to destroy everyone and everything. It came from the same place, and now we have to choose. Do we want to live in harmonious relationship with the whole universe (the word *universe* means, literally *'one song'*), or do we want to kill each other and destroy this beautiful planet in the process? We have to make this choice collectively, and soon. There is no one 'out there' who can make this choice on our behalf.

Radiation, we have discovered, cannot easily be localized. A nuclear explosion in Chernobyl contaminated the grass being grazed by sheep in the north of England, which affected the people eating them everywhere. Radiation has brought home to us just how closely inter–dependent we really are. We can no longer act in isolation and expect to be free of the consequences.

Interestingly, the internet is teaching us the same thing. I'm sure it is no coincidence that the internet has taken off with unstoppable momentum in recent years. Everybody has to be on the internet now, and nobody really knows why. It's a phenomenon that has a life of its own, and it is rapidly connecting everyone on the planet to everyone else, aided by the ubiquitous spread of the cellphone.

Communication channels are being put in place that have never existed before, so that information, and therefore power, cannot be controlled as they have been in the past. No person or government has managed to take control and rule the internet. We are literally creating a self–organizing nervous system across the entire planet at breathtaking speed, and, as far as we know, nothing quite like this has ever happened before.

One theory as to why there are so many humans on the planet at this time is that souls have chosen to incarnate now because a collective choice has to be made. Regardless of where we are born, we are connected to everybody else. The awareness of that connection is in the collective consciousness now. Perhaps everything is being put in place so that we can participate in the quantum leap in consciousness that is so urgently needed.

Resources

Ian Watson's audio recordings are available in mp3 format at: **www.ianwatsondownloads.com**

Information on Ian's self–healing workshops and retreats can be found at: **www.ianwatsonseminars.com**

Further information and supplies of the flower essences mentioned in this book are available via the following websites:

Bailey Flower Essences   www.baileyessences.com
Bach Flower Essences   www.healingherbs.co.uk
Australian Bush Flower Essences   www.ausflowers.com.au
Lightbringer Essences   www.lightbe.co.uk

U.K. distributors for all of the above essences and also for Ian Watson's book titles   www.healthlines.co.uk

Lightning Source UK Ltd.
Milton Keynes UK
06 December 2010